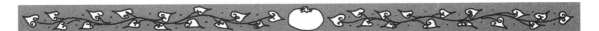

Suzanne Somers'
GET SKINNY
ON FABULOUS FOOD

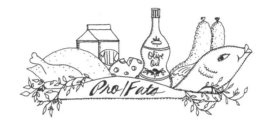

BY SUZANNE SOMERS

Illustrations by Leslie Hamel

Foreword by Diana Schwarzbein, M.D.

THREE RIVERS PRESS · NEW YORK

Grateful acknowledgment to Jeff Katz for photographs on pages 66, 107, 116, 119, 135, 151, 159, 163, 181, 187, 205

Published by Three Rivers Press, New York, New York.
Member of the Crown Publishing Group.

Random House, Inc. New York, Toronto, London, Sydney, Auckland
www.randomhouse.com

THREE RIVERS PRESS is a registered trademark and the Three Rivers Press colophon is a trademark of Random House, Inc.

Printed in the United States of America

Design by Debbie Glasserman and Lauren Dong

Library of Congress Cataloging-in-Publication Data
Somers, Suzanne
Suzanne Somers' get skinny on fabulous food / by Suzanne Somers :
illustrations by Leslie Hamel.
p.   cm.
1. Reducing diets—Recipes.   2. Sugar-free diet—Recipes.   I. Title.
RM222.2 S6553   1999   99-13372
613.2'5—dc21   CIP

ISBN 0-609-80237-2

10   9   8   7   6   5   4   3   2   1

First Paperback Edition

To my mother,
until we are together again.

Acknowledgments

There are so many to thank for their involvement in this project. At the top of the list is my daughter-in-law, Caroline Somers. It is inspiring to work alongside a great thinker. Caroline gathered research from nutritionists, endocrinologists, and various other sources for scientific data. Her enthusiasm kept me going in spite of my schedule overload and her attention to detail and correctness made this a better book. Caroline, your contribution was invaluable. Thank you, sweetheart.

My talented stepdaughter Leslie Hamel, working quietly and creatively at home, one day surprised me with pages of humorous and darling illustrations. "These are perfect," I told her, awed by her abilities. I am very lucky to have inherited two fabulous daughters whom I dearly love.

The team at Crown was once again supportive throughout the entire project: Chip Gibson, Andy Martin, Steve Ross, Wendy Schuman, and my talented and smart editor, Kristin Kiser. We had a great working relationship of mutual support and literary resonance. Thank you, Kristin.

Al Lowman, my super agent, was, as always, probing and interested. He's never been a "take-the-commission-and-run" kind of guy. He's with me all the way, reading, questioning, offering suggestions, faxing title ideas back and forth, going to bat when necessary. Thanks, Al. This is our third together, let's do a lot more.

To my lawyer, Marc Chamlin, thank you for your expertise and smart thinking.

Jeff Katz, my favorite photographer, took the cover and insert photos. As always, Jeff and his team worked long, hard, arduous days climbing up and down the hills of my desert property carrying loads of cables, filters, sun umbrellas, and cases and cases of camera equipment. Jeff was always upbeat and cheerful, his only agenda being great pictures . . . and they *are* beautiful! The food looks like it could jump off the page into your mouth. A big thanks and gratitude to Jeff Katz and his wonderful team: Victor Voghossian, John Coier, Sheri Harbison, and Andrew Strauss.

Donna Glennon was my set stylist, and once again was at her perfectionist best. It was Donna and her team who carried the bed up the hillside to take the "Never thought I'd be so happy *not* to have a *roof over my head*" photo. Donna works tirelessly in her quest to get the perfect picture.

I so appreciate you, Donna, and also your talented and happy team, Rio Bininger and Sylvia Medellin.

Bryan Wark did the flowers. I admire restraint, and when he felt it appropriate Bryan knew when a single flower was the perfect touch, even going so far as to climb my palm trees to get date berries to complete the New Year's Eve table setting. Thank you for your talent, Bryan.

Samantha Degen is always my stylist of choice. I sent her into my closet and she found things I forgot were there. She knows

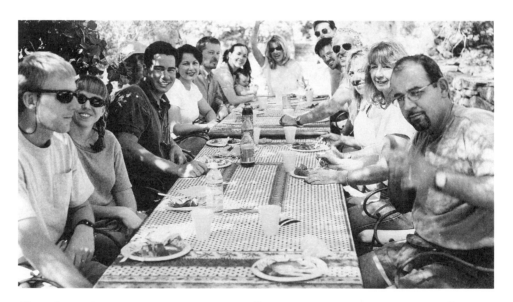

The photo shoot team enjoying our Somersized lunch under the Palo Verde tree at our desert home. Andrew Strauss, Sheri Harbison, Rio Bininger, Sylvia Medellin, Bryan Wark, my daughter-in-law Caroline Somers, Violet, me, Jeff Katz (my favorite photographer), my son Bruce Somers, Alan, Debra Murray, Trish Gardener, and Victor Voghossian.

the right dress or the perfect sweater for each photo. "No jewelry," she often says. And she is right. (Unless, of course, it's my Suzanne Somers' Collection of Jewelry on the Home Shopping Network!)

Cathy Highland did my hair and makeup for the photos, often applying hair spray while I was in the kitchen making Turkey Shiitake Mushroom Soup or some other yummy concoction. I trusted her talent and for several of the photos I never even looked in a mirror because I knew she'd make it look right.

Trish Gardener, who has looked after my home for many years, was invaluable in helping all of us.

Sue Balmforth was a true friend. Sue owns the most wonderful vintage antique store in Venice, California, called Bountiful. "Take anything you want," she told me, so I did! EVEN HER BED! Yes, she gave me her own bed and slept on the floor until we brought it back. Thank you for your generosity, Sue.

Ken Brown graciously gave me five of his favorite recipes from Urban Epicuria, the gourmet take-away storefront in West Hollywood. Many of his recipes fall into the Somersize category. Thank you, Ken.

Mary Schuck, thank you for your beautiful cover design, and thank you, too, to Amy Boorstein, Lauren Dong, and Jane Searle for shepherding this book through production.

To Felipe and Lisbet of El Mirasol Restaurant in our beloved desert. We loved the delicious catered lunches during the photo shoot.

And my team in the office . . . Anka, Kristin, and, of course, Marsha. They are the ones who do all the running around, pick-ups, deliveries, FedExes, faxes, typing, and suggesting much more! You are the best.

Thanks to Bruce, Camelia, and Violet for their participation. Bruce, my darling son, put his flourishing business on hold for a few days to baby-sit so Caroline could help me cook. And thank you to two of my granddaughters, Camelia and Violet, for letting us dress you up in my white antique linen and lace baby dress collection.

Alan, my great husband, who is always there for me with ideas and encouragement and, of course, to make the best deals. I love you! We make a great team.

Debra Murray, my food stylist on Home Shopping, who cooked, tested, cooked some more, and tested yet even more for months and months. Thank you, Debra, for your hard work and dedication.

And finally, my chief source of information came from Dr. Diana Schwarzbein, the renowned endocrinologist from Santa Barbara. Dr. Schwarzbein is in the vanguard of new medicine and gave me profound information regarding diet and health. Her understanding of food and its effects on hormones and the delicate balance our bodies require to stay disease-free and healthy will change your life as it has mine. Her foreword has invaluable information regarding a new approach to eating for a long and healthy life. More information can be obtained from her book *The Schwarzbein Principle,* by Diana Schwarzbein, M.D. Thank you, Diana. Your brilliance astounds me.

And thanks to all of you who bought and embraced the principles of my book *Eat Great, Lose Weight.* It is because of you I wrote this second book. You wanted more information and more recipes. Every one of the thousands of letters you sent telling me how much weight you have lost, how easy you find the program, and how it has changed your life makes me happier than I can describe. This plan works for me and I feel blessed to be able to share it with you.

Thank you all and enjoy *Getting Skinny on Fabulous Food!*

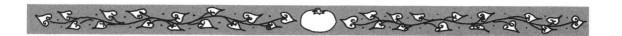

Contents

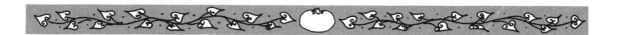

Foreword

Knowing what I know today, it is still hard for me to accept that between 1981 and 1990, while I was in nine years of medical training, my instructors were teaching me and everyone else in medical training that a low-fat diet was the way to prevent obesity, diabetes, and heart attacks. My instructors stressed the "fact" that eating fat not only made you fat but also caused a host of health problems. These professors spoke of hundreds of studies that they said proved that fat was indeed the culprit in creating a national epidemic of obesity, diabetes, and heart disease.

Countless magazines and newspapers shared the results of these studies with the public. These studies fueled a frenzy outside of medical schools as people got caught up in trying to lose weight and prevent heart disease by reducing or eliminating fat from their diets. And the short-term effects of eating less fat and more carbohydrates seemed to indicate that people could lose weight and decrease their cholesterol by eating this way.

But these studies proved to be wrong. This may come as a surprise to you, but cutting back fat from your diet and filling up on carbohydrates may actually cause you to gain weight in the long run, can increase your cholesterol level, and can set you down a path of what I call "accelerated metabolic aging." A low-fat diet eaten over a long period of time actually deprives humans of the nutrients they need to regenerate healthy cells, which can lead to disease and early death. The studies referred to by my professors in medical school only took into account the short term. There were—and are—no long-term studies that show a low-fat, high-carbohydrate diet maintains weight over the long run and prevents illness.

Since leaving medical school I have radically changed how I think about nutrition and health. No longer do I believe that fat is evil and carbohydrates are good. From my own clinical research with thousands of patients, I now have a better understanding of what we all need to eat to control our weight and prevent disease. I no longer advocate a low-fat diet, but instead teach all of my patients how to balance their meals, like Suzanne Somers does so well in *Get Skinny on Fabulous Food*. Suzanne understands what I came to discover after leaving medical school—that the secret to weight loss and maintenance lies in controlling the amount of the hormone insulin that is released into our bloodstream after a meal. And the secret to preventing disease is to make sure we eat foods that can rebuild our cells and keep them strong.

Over the years I have come to understand how vitally important it is that people stop eating a low-fat, high-carbohydrate diet and start combining their food properly. This understanding started when I took a job at a medical clinic in Santa Barbara, California. I was hired to reestablish a diabetes program there. I would spend a full hour with each diabetic patient, obtaining a detailed history. These were type II diabetics, which accounts for 98 percent of diabetes. With this type of diabetes, the body produces insulin, the hormone responsible for getting sugar into the cells, but the patients' cells do not respond well to insulin—they are what is called insulin resistant.

As I listened to the patients' stories, it was clear that they were very upset that instead of getting better after seeking medical help, they were steadily getting worse. They told

me that they had started off eating the American Diabetes Association (ADA) diet, which is a low-fat, high-carbohydrate diet. They checked their blood sugars regularly. When they came back to the doctor, the doctor would tell them that they had not been compliant—if they had been, their blood sugars, cholesterol, and weight would be better. Imagine how you'd feel if you'd done precisely what the doctor ordered and not only did you get worse, the doctor as much as called you a liar!

The next therapeutic step was to add in one of the sugar-lowering drugs while continuing to follow the same diet.

During their next follow-up visits they were again told that they must be noncompliant because they were not getting well. A lot of them were then switched from pills to insulin injections. And you guessed it, they still did not get better (remember, these patients are insulin resistant). And if the doctor did believe that they were following their diet, the fact that they were not getting better was attributed to genetic problems and they were still put on insulin injections.

You can see how frustrating this must have been for them. I certainly felt their frustration and anger when I heard these stories. And then I realized I had two choices. I could continue with the same standard treatment regimens that these patients were already on or the patients and I would have to come up with a new treatment plan.

I gave each of these patients a choice. Every one of them wanted to come up with something different, so we started by collecting baseline data. I had them write down everything they put in their mouths. I had them check their blood sugars six times a day, before and after their meals. First thing in the morning I had patients measure their blood sugar. It was always normal. Then they had the breakfast recommended by the ADA, typically a bowl of cereal with nonfat milk, a banana, and a glass of fruit juice. Nondiabetics eating this breakfast would experience only a ten- to twenty-point rise in their blood sugar. But after this high-carbohydrate, low-fat ADA-recommended breakfast, my patients would watch their blood sugar soar—up between 100 and 200 points, ten times the normal blood sugar response.

It had to be the diet that made their blood sugar levels soar, but why? And then it suddenly hit me—their blood sugar rose dramatically because we were feeding them hidden sugars: hidden sugars in the form of carbohydrates. All carbohydrates are broken down into sugar by the body during digestion, whether they are in the form of grains, starches, dairy, fruits, or sweets. By recommending a high-carbohydrate diet, we were asking diabetics to eat sugar.

After seeing these patients' blood sugar levels rise so dramatically after meals, I was convinced that the ADA diet was wrong. Though it was professionally a tough decision for me, I had to turn my back on the ADA-approved diet and conventional learning. The new clinical evidence was too strong. All of my type II diabetic patients reported the same results: the ADA diet made their blood sugar skyrocket.

Now the real process began. If not the ADA diet, what *should* these patients be eating? I started with the premise that it should be as few carbohydrates as possible, since they were converted to sugar. So that left proteins, fats, and nonstarchy vegetables. However, I asked them to keep their fat intake to a minimum because type II diabetics have the highest risk of heart disease of any patient population. Limiting fat seemed wise since I still believed at that time that eating fat caused heart disease.

The most important clinical question was: Could we get the patients' blood sugars lower while still keeping heart disease at a low level?

One week later the first group of patients returned for an evaluation. I looked at the blood sugar numbers they had recorded. Their progress was astounding. But the ones who had improved the most were the "cheaters." On their own, with the help of their home sugar-measuring devices, they were seeing that their blood sugar levels were improving when they ate more fat with their meals. Soon they were eating even more mayonnaise, butter, cheese, eggs, and steak. What a delight, after months or years of shredded wheat and nonfat milk!

By *cutting down* on carbohydrates and *eating fats*, they were *losing* weight! For a type II diabetic, losing weight is an almost impossible feat. But these patients were eating fats and losing body fat and it did not end with just losing weight. Everything was improving. They felt satiated and their energy improved. Their cholesterol levels were improving. And because their cholesterol levels were getting better and not worse—believe me, I was monitoring this closely—it encouraged me and my patients to continue this regimen.

My biggest fear—that I would treat their diabetes but increase their risk of heart attacks—proved groundless. Why? Because weight gain around the middle of the body, high blood pressure, high blood sugars, and high cholesterol levels are all risk factors for heart disease and every one of these conditions was improving!

So how did treating diabetics with this diet plan change how I treat all my patients? Because I started to look at our similarities as humans. We all have mouths, stomachs, small intestines, portal veins, and livers. We all digest carbohydrates into sugars by using the same enzymes. We all secrete the same hormones in response to the food that we are eating. Our livers all have the capacity to turn sugars into fat and cholesterol. Our bodies all function the same.

And that is when I started testing my hypothesis on other patients who were not diabetic. It worked for them, too!

I was more astonished with each passing day. Every single patient thrived as he or she adopted this more balanced eating plan— fewer carbohydrates and all the proteins, fats, and nonstarchy vegetables they wanted. Those who needed to lose weight did so effortlessly. Those who were already in good shape found themselves with more energy.

While I was watching my patients get healthy while eating fat, it made me realize that I had never met anyone who followed a low-fat diet who was as healthy as my patients were becoming. Well, I thought, maybe it was just that those people I saw came for treatment of some problem. Maybe there were many healthy low-fat dieters out there who never needed a doc-

tor. Or, and this is a frightening thought, were they only healthy temporarily because they hadn't eaten that way long enough for the damage to their bodies to show up?

This was when I conducted a thorough search of the medical literature and discovered that there was not a single long-term study that proved that a low-fat, high-carbohydrate diet was beneficial to our health. However, I did find thirty years' worth of basic science studies that proved that high insulin levels were linked to heart disease, high blood pressure, excessive increase in body fat, and many other problems. This is when I concluded that the population studies were not as important in determining how to be healthy as basic science was. Population studies take a segment of the population, follow it for a few years, and try to come up with conclusions. The variability involved in population studies makes this an almost impossible task. On the contrary, basic science is the study of how the body actually works in physiological terms. Basic science does not change greatly. However, every time you turn around the population studies are telling you how to eat differently. If we just stick to science everyone would stay on a balanced eating program consisting of healthy, nutritious foods, the kind of program Suzanne Somers advocates in her books.

You have seen how we have debunked the myth that eating fat makes you fat by actually looking at basic human physiology, which proves that increased insulin levels cause weight gain. Now let's go ahead and debunk another myth—that consuming excess calories causes weight gain.

A calorie is simply the amount of energy required to raise one gram of water one degree Celsius. Proteins and carbohydrates each have four calories per gram. Fat has nine calories per gram. Therefore, fat is more than twice as fattening as proteins and carbohydrates, right? Wrong!

What happens in a test tube is not the same as what happens in your body. In your body, a carbohydrate snack must be used for immediate energy or it is stored as fat. But if the snack is protein and fat, the food is used first to replace cells, enzymes, and hormones that are made up of proteins and fats, which leaves fewer leftover calories to be stored around your middle.

After I discovered this, it became clear to me why my patients were able to consume *more* calories and *more* fat and still not gain weight. Once again, all signs were pointing to hormone changes in the body as the reason why people lose or gain weight. When insulin levels and their effects are higher, people are more prone to storing fuel as fat.

But I still had more work to do to convince my nondiabetic patients that eating fats was essential. They proved to themselves through experience that eating fat would not make them fat, but they were still worried that consuming more fat and cholesterol would lead to heart disease. So I began telling them how cholesterol and fat are essential to health and life. They are used by the body as building materials, and they need to come from the food you eat. Fat and cholesterol don't cause heart disease; in fact, you must eat them to *avoid* heart disease and early death. The more good fats you eat, the healthier you will be.

Look at the good that cholesterol accomplishes in your body:

1. Essential for brain function
2. Forms insulation around nerves to keep electrical impulses moving
3. Forms membranes inside cells
4. Provides important structures in cell membranes
5. Keeps cell membranes permeable
6. Helps prevent mood swings
7. Maintains a healthy immune system
8. Makes important hormones
9. Stabilizes neurotransmitters

I explain to my patients that the body is constantly breaking down cells and building them up again. Dietary fats play a key role in this replenishing process. Like cholesterol deprivation, fat deprivation disrupts all the biochemical processes of your metabolism. It would be impossible to list all the health problems that can occur as a result of depriving your body of fat, but here are a few signs and symptoms:

1. Brittle nails
2. Carbohydrate and stimulant craving
3. Constipation
4. Dry, limp, thinning hair
5. Infertility
6. Insomnia
7. Loss of lean body mass and fat gain around the middle
8. Mood disorders
9. Scaly, itchy skin

The solution to overcoming these conditions and avoiding many more is to eat good dietary fats. Fats found in nature are healthy. Saturated, monounsaturated, and polyunsaturated fats are all natural fats and therefore good for you. Your diet should be rich in fat and cholesterol, which can come from a wide variety of foods, such as avocados, butter, eggs, red meat, chicken, shellfish, fish, olives, tofu, nuts, and seeds.

To summarize, let's take a quick look at "conventional wisdom," errors touted by everyone from women's magazines to the ADA, and compare it to what really happens in your body:

Conventional Wisdom: Eating fat makes your cholesterol rise, and puts you in heart-attack country.

The Truth: The high insulin levels created by a high-carbohydrate, low-fat diet cause plaque to be deposited in your arteries. Build enough plaque and you've built a heart attack. Eating fats and cholesterol lowers insulin levels and switches off the body's production of cholesterol, protecting you from heart attacks.

Conventional Wisdom: Risk of high blood pressure (hypertension) is increased by eating fat.

The Truth: Again, insulin is the real culprit. Without fat, insulin levels rise higher in the blood, which leads to other factors that cause high blood pressure.

Conventional Wisdom: The low-fat, high-carbohydrate diet for diabetics makes patients healthier.

The Truth: Type II diabetics are insulin resistant. Eating a low-fat, high-carbohydrate diet increases their insulin resistance. Patients get better on a balanced plan of protein, fats, nonstarchy vegetables, and limited carbohydrates.

Conventional Wisdom: A low-fat diet prevents cancer. A high-fat diet causes cancer.

The Truth: Cancer cells grow best when insulin levels are high, just the climate created by the low-fat, high-carbohydrate diet. Dietary fat increases a healthy immune system and gives the body key components to fight cancer cells.

You now see why I am on the fat bandwagon. Eating fat isn't making us fat—it's the low-fat, high-carbohydrate diet that raises our insulin levels. There are some other factors that raise insulin levels, too, both directly and indirectly. These include dieting, stress, lack of exercise, caffeine, alcohol, aspartame, tobacco, steroids, stimulants and other recreational drugs, excessive and/or unnecessary thyroid replacement therapy, and all over-the-counter and prescription drugs. These insulin-stimulating factors have defined the lifestyle habits that have prevailed over the last twenty years in this country and parallel the rise in the incidence of disease during the same period of time. A more complete exploration of the science as well as the nutritional and lifestyle program I recommend to my patients can be found in *The Schwarzbein Principle* (Health Communications, Inc., 1999).

It has been a delight to come to know Suzanne Somers as a patient, friend, and co-crusader for healthier eating habits. In *Get Skinny on Fabulous Food,* you will find practical, easy-to-understand advice about eating proteins and fats while limiting carbohydrates. I am thrilled to see someone with Suzanne's exposure finally getting the right message out to people. We must reverse the common thinking that a low-fat, high-carbohydrate diet is the key to health and weight loss. While her thoughts on food combining are outside the scope of my own research, her information regarding the health benefits of adopting a lifestyle that lowers insulin levels are completely accurate. Those who follow Suzanne's advice by adhering to a diet full of proteins, fats, and vegetables will create a healthy, leaner, and more vigorous body.

DIANA SCHWARZBEIN, M.D.
Santa Barbara, California

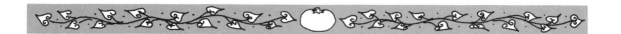

Introduction

Okay, all you "Somersizers," more than a million of you have discovered how to stay slim, healthy, and energetic with my easy-to-follow program, "Eat Great, Lose Weight." Indeed, "Somersizing" has swept the nation, teaching former dieters in despair how to eat incredible, rich foods in abundant portions while the unwanted pounds effortlessly melt away. My enthusiasm for this program grows each day as the letters continue to pour in with one success story after the next. Because of the overwhelming response from people all over the country, I feel compelled to share *more* information about the importance of adopting this lifestyle, a lifestyle that allows you to enjoy food, rather than fear it; a lifestyle that allows *you* to be in control of your weight rather than your weight being in control of you; a lifestyle that includes total fitness, from the inside out, where food becomes your friend and your partner in helping you achieve optimum health.

Get Skinny on Fabulous Food, my second book in the Somersizing series, further dispels the myth that fat is the enemy. In the past decade we have been bombarded with message after message that not only will fat make you fat, but it will lead to disease and early death. In response, our country has exploded into a fat-free craze that has exceeded the popularity of the Beatles. Fat-free cookies, fat-free cakes, fat-free ice cream . . . but can these fat-free treats actually keep you slim and healthy? Absolutely not! Products loaded with sugar, white flour, hydrogenated oils, and chemicals and preservatives that replace *real fats* are harmful to your figure and your general health. The fat-free *craze* has developed into a *craziness* leading Americans to believe that Olestra, a fake fat recently approved by the FDA, is a healthy alternative to real fat. Never mind the side effects of the synthetic food—abdominal cramping and loose stool syndrome!

Don't be fooled by manufacturers trying to make a buck off your "fear of fat." The news is in—and the news is great! There is no need to be afraid of fat. Over a million of you on my program have been losing weight by indulging in foods like eggs, cream, meat, and cheese without increasing your cholesterol levels. It sounds too good to be true, but it's based on important physiological findings.

Get Skinny on Fabulous Food includes medical validation from leading endocrinologist Diana Schwarzbein, M.D., who argues that the fear of fat is not grounded in scientific fact. If you skipped over the foreword she wrote for this book, I urge you to go back and read it. Her clinical research reinforces that eating fat will not make you fat. Fat is your friend. I want to shout it from the mountaintops: "You can eat fat and it doesn't make you fat!" Furthermore, Dr. Schwarzbein warns that almost entirely eliminating foods containing cholesterol and fat from your diet can actually accelerate metabolic aging, leading to increased risk of disease and death.

In this book you'll read astounding findings showing that many young women in their twenties and thirties fit into a frightening profile. They exercise multiple times a week, they eat a low-fat, high-carbohydrate diet, and they drink mostly water and diet sodas. One would think they would be the picture of health. But medical analysis shows these women have the metabolic age and bone density typically seen in eighty-year-olds! The lack of fat and protein in their diet has set them on a premature path toward osteoporosis and early disease.

Dr. Schwarzbein also provides compelling information that avoiding fat disrupts our hormonal system. We must eat fat in order to produce essential hormones. And we must produce hormones in order to replace and re-create healthy cells. Eliminating fat from our diets can actually cause a halt in our hormone production, which in turn causes cell abnormalities. When cell abnormalities develop, we are most prone to disease. The importance of including dietary fats becomes apparent when you see the link: disease sets in when healthy hormone replacement is halted from a lack of real fats in our diet. Menopausal women are especially at risk because their hormonal system is already in turmoil with decreased estrogen levels. Therefore, not only does Dr. Schwarzbein support ingesting Somersize favorites like butter, sour cream, and sausage, but she asserts one *must* include real fats as part of a healthy diet. Her research shows the more good fats one eats, the healthier one becomes. Not only is Somersizing a delicious way to eat, it is also a safe and effective way to lose weight. Eating this way is essential to our health.

In *Get Skinny on Fabulous Food,* I'll give you a short recap of my Somersize program, showing how you can eat formerly forbidden foods in proper combinations and still lose weight. Plus I'll unveil the true enemy—*sugar* and foods that are immediately converted to sugar upon ingestion, such as white flour, potatoes, and white rice. By eliminating these foods, in addition to alcohol and caffeine, you can enjoy all those rich treats while staying healthy, energetic, and lean. Yes, you can get skinny on fats!

You'll also see dramatic "before and after" pictures from many of the men and women who have had such incredible success on this program. And I've included excerpts from the emotional letters they have sent to me, detailing the difference Somersizing has made in their lives. They share their stories of how before Somersizing they had tried every diet known to man *and* woman; how they would lose the weight and then gain it all back, including a few extra pounds. They talk about their depression and constant hunger. When they first found my program they thought it sounded too good to be true. But they tried it, and it worked. Now they tell me their energy has never been better and that they lost the weight without ever going hungry. They can't believe they've gotten down to their goal weight while eating cheese and steak and butter and sour cream! I spoke with a woman named Lynn Thorpe who went from 407 pounds down to 174 with *Eat Great, Lose Weight.* She is astounded at the difference it's made in her life. She has a whole new confidence. She says she walks differently. Men look at her. And this time

she knows it's staying off for good because this isn't a diet—it's a new outlook on life.

Get Skinny on Fabulous Food also explores the emotional side of making bad eating choices. Why do we eat when we're depressed or stressed or feeling insecure? Why do we use comfort food as our friend, our lover, and our nurturer? Achieving optimum health works from the inside out. When we make the commitment to make a change in our life, the results can be staggering, both physically and emotionally.

Part of Somersizing is realizing that food is no longer the enemy. Now that I know *how* to eat, I no longer have to feel guilty about it. I have grown to value and appreciate what food means to me. In fact, my most cherished times revolve around food and family. That's why I've included a very personal section called "Family Dinners" to show you how I connect with those I love around the dinner table and the importance of that ritual in our lives.

And you've asked for more recipes. *Get Skinny on Fabulous Food* includes more than 130 new favorites with full-color photographs of my exciting appetizers, salads,

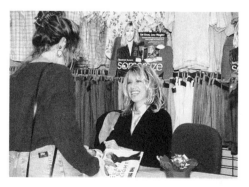

On the promotion trail for Somersizing.

soups, side dishes, and entrées. You'll love losing weight on Milanese beef with sautéed onions and mushrooms in a port wine sauce, succulent pork chops with delectable pan drippings, herb-crusted halibut with tomatoes and basil, and perfectly roasted leg of lamb. And don't forget my signature desserts, including cappuccino chocolate-chunk cheesecake, mountain of lemon meringue pie, and raspberry crème brûlée.

I got skinny on fabulous food. I know the program works. It's worked for me and hundreds of thousands of others. It's easy to follow. There is no counting calories. There is no counting fat grams. There is no depri-

vation. There is no guilt. I promise you will never go hungry. The food is unbelievable. The food is real. And, most important, the program is medically sound. You'll not only look great on the outside, you'll adopt a new lifestyle that will keep you young and healthy on the inside. It is urgent that you eat this way. This book contains vital information that goes far beyond weight loss. Somersizing is the next step in understanding how to achieve our maximum potential; how to take control of our diet, our physique, our physical health, and our emotional well-being. It can happen for you, too. Read on, then start today . . . and *Get Skinny on Fabulous Food*.

Part One

A NEW WAY

OF LIFE

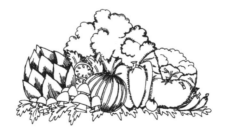

ONE

Diets—The Ultimate Empty Promise

If you've ever had a problem with your weight, you've probably tried one diet after the next. At first you stick to it diligently. You're excited because you really think this is going to be the one to solve all your problems. You count and measure and deprive yourself of eating the foods you love, all in the quest to become thin. The pounds drop slowly . . . too slowly. Irritability increases because you're hungry and cranky. As the days pass you're upset because you feel surrounded by thin people who seem to be able to eat whatever they want while you hold the dressing on the salad and eat a boring chicken breast with no sauce. You watch those fat grams, keep those calories down. You're miserable because your whole life seems to revolve around what you can eat or, rather, what you *can't* eat. But you stick to it, because nothing would make you feel more attractive and healthier than a new slim figure.

After two solid weeks of dieting, you pass by the open cupboard and notice a bag of Pepperidge Farm cookies that has been left opened. You go to roll down the top of the bag to keep them fresh, but first you peek inside. Oh, the smell. There is one broken cookie left on the top row. You *can't* eat it. Well, you *could,* but you shouldn't. But it just looks so messy having that one broken cookie resting on the white ruffled piece of paper. You decide you really should clean up that bag and remove that top piece of paper. You bite your fingernail and rationalize that since you've been so good, it would be okay to treat yourself to one minuscule crumb. You go for it, and your mouth explodes. Oh, what you've been missing! One little cookie crumb instantly makes your willpower crumble. It's okay, you convince yourself. It's not gonna kill you to eat the rest of that one measly little broken cookie. You look to see if any family members are nearby. The coast is clear, so you pop the delectable treat into your mouth. It's crunchy and sweet. The chocolate is rich and delicious.

Since you've already blown your diet, before you know it you've removed the white paper and are digging into the second row for another cookie. After one and a half cookies you decide you might as well have another to completely satisfy your craving so you can get back on track tomorrow. You inhale cookie number two, licking your fingers to get every morsel. You go to close the bag and realize there's just one cookie left in the row, and it looks entirely too lonely sitting there by itself. You down it and remove the second piece of white paper. Now you're full, but there is only one row left in the entire bag—and having them around may tempt you to cheat again—so you polish off the rest of the bag and hide the evidence in the trash can.

Then comes the guilt. "I shouldn't have done it." Then comes the bloating. "I feel sick to my stomach." Then comes the despair. "I'll never lose this weight." Then comes the depression. "What difference does it make. I'm gonna be fat forever." So much for the diet. In a short time you gain back all the weight you lost and a few extra pounds on top of that. Then it's time to scour the fashion magazines and find the new diet that *promises* to help you lose the weight and keep it off for good.

Diets—the ultimate *empty promise* perpetuating the same cycle over and over again. We've all been victims of yo-yo dieting. We stick to some diets longer than others, but c'mon, just how much cabbage soup can a person eat? Let's face it . . . most diets fail because they are based on deprivation, and after depriving yourself for a period of time, you will eventually want to reward yourself. During the reward time, you will probably gain back all the weight, plus more. Staggering statistics show that 95 percent of us who go on diets gain back all the weight. Something is terribly wrong!

So how do we beat the statistics? I'm happy to say I have finally figured it out. If you read my first book, you heard about my battle with dieting and how a trip to France in 1992 and an introduction to food combining changed everything for me. I stopped dieting on plain, boring, unsatisfying food and started eating rich, delicious meals full of flavor and, yes . . . *fat*. I got skinny on fat and realized I would never have to diet again. By eating a balanced diet including fresh fruit, vegetables, whole grains, butter, cheese, eggs, meat, and even cream, I went from 130 pounds down to 116, the amount I weighed as a teenager. And because I give my body real foods, my hunger is satisfied and I am meeting my body's nutritional needs. In the last six years my weight has not fluctuated by more than five pounds. This is not another diet full of empty promises . . . it's a remarkable program that has helped over a million people to lose weight and gain energy—Somersizing.

MESSING WITH YOUR METABOLISM

Why do diets fail time and time again? First of all, diets are about deprivation. We simply don't get to eat enough food, or enough of the right kinds of food, to satisfy our bodies' needs. Let's look at what happens when you restrict your calories from, for example, 1,500 to 1,000 calories a day. Since your body is used to running on 1,500 calories, it must make up for the missing fuel source by burning off first your glycogen and protein stores and then your fat reserves to provide you with enough energy to get through the day. This initial burning of fuel is why you will lose weight when you cut your calories. (Glycogen is stored with water, and therefore weighs more than fat. The scale may reflect a substantial weight loss due mostly to the loss of water, not fat. That's what the term "water weight" means.) But the human body is a remarkably complicated and adaptable machine. As your glycogen and protein stores are being depleted, your metabolism will actually slow down to keep you from starving to death. It's a survival instinct. Your body adapts to survive on 1,000 calories, or less fuel than it needed before. Plus, this new lower metabolism means you have a slower-running machine—quite simply, less energy to get you through the day, leaving you tired and listless.

It is at this point that your weight usually plateaus. But it gets even worse. Your body recognizes it's not getting enough food, so it starts to store away a portion of the fuel. It may use 800 calories for fuel and store 200 as fat for later use. So even though you're still eating like a bird, sticking faithfully to your diet, you're exhausted from a lack of energy and you're actually gaining a couple of pounds! That's when frustration sets in and we attack the bag of cookies in the cupboard like a cheetah on antelope.

Here's the worst part. You now have an even lower metabolism than before you started the diet, so your body needs fewer calories to survive. When you go back to eating the way you used to at 1,500 calories a day, your body will have an excess of fuel because it has learned to survive on 800 calories a day. Therefore you have an additional 700 calories that will be stored as fat for later use. That's why you gain *all* the weight back and probably a little extra because of your new lower metabolism.

Up and down the diet roller coaster we go. Appetite suppressants create the same scenario. Diet pills kill our appetite, so we eat less and resist fatty foods we've been trained to think are off limits. Eating fewer calories starts the weight loss process, but our bodies adjust to eating this smaller amount of food by lowering the metabolism to keep us from starving to death. Once again, the body's natural survival instinct kicks in. As soon as you go off the diet pills, your appetite will return . . . and so will all the pounds you lost and then some, because of your new lower metabolism.

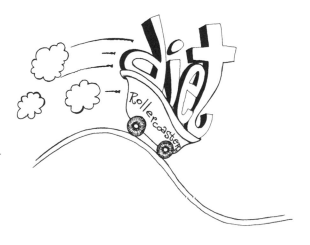

For those of you who got duped into the Phen-Fen trend, you now know exactly what I'm talking about. You probably lost a substantial amount of weight as long as you were taking the drugs, but when you tried to get off them, the weight crept back on quickly. Phen-Fen was meant only for the truly obese, not for someone wanting to lose a couple of dress sizes. Thank goodness those dangerous drugs are now off the market. But in their wake they've left thousands of dieters with a messed-up metabolism that is in need of repair.

REPROGRAM YOUR METABOLISM

Somersizing is a lifestyle . . . a whole new way of eating that will change your thinking about losing weight and gaining energy. The plan is simple. I will teach you to eat real food—and plenty of it—in a way that reprograms your metabolism to burn fat and give you a constant source of energy.

Level One is the weight loss portion of the program. I'll explain the specifics later on in this book, but here's the basic overview. First I eliminate a small list of foods that wreak havoc on our systems, like sugar, white flour, and potatoes, and then I eat normal everyday foods in combinations that aid in digestion and weight control. In order to increase your metabolism, you must eat food! I eat whenever I am hungry. I do not skimp on portions. I eat until I am full, and I never skip meals.

Here's how it works. I have taken readily available foods and categorized them into four Somersized Food Groups:

Pro/Fats: Includes proteins like meat, poultry, fish, and eggs, and fats in their natural state, like oil, butter, cream, and cheese.

Veggies: Includes a host of low-starch, fresh vegetables from artichokes to peppers to zucchini and more.

Carbos: Includes whole-grain pastas, cereals, breads, beans, and nonfat dairy products.

Fruit: Includes a huge variety of fresh fruit from apples to peaches to tangerines and more.

The group of foods I eliminate are called "Funky Foods," because they don't fit into any of the four Somersized Food Groups:

Funky Foods: Includes sugars, highly starchy foods, caffeine, and alcohol. (You will find complete lists of all of these groups in the following chapters.)

Here are the basic guidelines of Level One, the weight loss portion of my program.

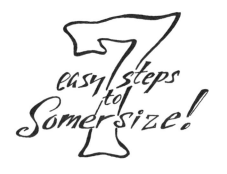

1. Eliminate all FUNKY FOODS.
2. Eat FRUIT alone, on an empty stomach.
3. Eat PRO/FATS with VEGGIES.
4. Eat CARBOS with VEGGIES.
5. Keep PRO/FATS separate from CARBOS.
6. Wait three hours between meals if switching from a PRO/FATS meal to a CARBOS meal, or vice versa.
7. Do not skip meals. Eat at least three meals a day, and eat until you feel satisfied and comfortably full.

Seven easy steps. That's it. I mean it! As long as you follow all of the Level One guidelines, you may eat until you are full and still lose weight. You probably don't believe me, right? You probably think later in the book I will reveal that you have to mix powders or take pills or count calories and fat grams or buy special Somersized prepackaged foods or fast for the first week. Nope. Just follow these seven easy steps, enjoy delicious, flavorful foods without ever going hungry, and you will reprogram your metabolism to help you lose weight and gain energy.

How? Somersizing promotes *hormonal balance,* which is the key to achieving your ideal body weight and optimum health. Foods high in sugar and refined carbohydrates cause hormonal imbalance, which leads to weight gain. Remember puberty? We didn't change our eating habits, yet overnight we suddenly started gaining weight. The reason is because our hormones were changing. The same is true for menopausal women; suddenly there is a thickness around the hips while the body's hormonal levels are in a state of flux.

Somersizing teaches us to eat foods that *balance our hormones;* foods like protein, fats, and vegetables low in starch. If you take away only one piece of information from this book, it should be this: *It is not fat and calories that cause weight gain . . . it is hormonal imbalance.*

It's such a breeze and a delight to eat this way. Take a look at what you might eat in a sample day. You could start your morning with a piece of fruit, then have a shower and follow up with a bowl of whole-grain cereal with nonfat milk. For lunch you might choose a large Caesar salad with chicken and a side of sautéed vegetables sprinkled with Parmesan cheese. In the afternoon you could decide to snack on fresh fruit or a hard-boiled egg. And for dinner, try a green salad with blue cheese dressing, a big juicy steak, and a side of broccoli . . . covered with cheese sauce if you like! No deprivation here.

The key is the combination of foods we choose at every meal. Your perfectly combined steak dinner could be instantly destroyed by eating a plate of fruit for dessert. Fruit should not be combined with other foods because it causes gas and bloating and may upset the digestive process of other foods. In addition, we keep the proteins and fats separate from the carbohydrates—notice there's no rice, pasta, or potato with that steak. But you do enjoy whole-grain carbos, which are especially great in the morning, with nonfat dairy products. What a perfect energy boost for the beginning of the day!

My Dear Friend,

Not knowing how to prepare deliciously healthy foods to work *for* me rather than *against* me has always been something my mind couldn't grasp. I was under the misconception that I had to eat as little as 600 calories a day in order to become thin. The more I obsessed about finding the right diet the larger I became; I had blossomed to a lonely *407* pounds! My self-esteem diminished to the point of wondering how I could ever end this vicious cycle; I was sinking. A couple of years ago I was watching you on TV. Dear Suzanne, little did I know the key I had prayed for was right in front of me. You were talking about starting a new way of life by changing eating habits. I listened, but didn't react till the next day when again I was flipping channels and there you were. I ordered your product, hoping that just maybe this would finally be the key to take this beautiful person out of this ugly body. I didn't open your book right away and even debated with myself if this really could work. But this little voice kept telling me don't wait. So I grabbed my shopping list & proceeded forward.

I wish for others to grab hold of your words, so they can truly teach their children a better way of life; and they don't go through the pain and suffering of crying themselves to sleep from this terrible disease called obesity.

If I ever see you, my dear friend, I'll give you the biggest hug for putting this great discovery out as my lifeline.

Now 174 pounds, I have a happier Heart, Mind & most of all . . . BODY.

With the utmost admiration and affection,
Lynn Thorpe

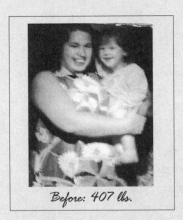
Before: 407 lbs.

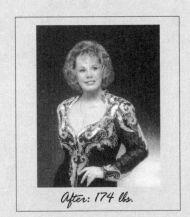
After: 174 lbs.

Overall, we get an excellent balance of foods—plenty of fresh fruit and vegetables to provide fiber, vitamins, and minerals; whole-grain carbohydrates for energy and additional fiber; and the protein and fat from meat and dairy products that is essential to our good health. By eating *real* foods instead of processed and refined foods, we are supplying our body with the building materials it needs to keep us healthy and youthful—not just on the outside, but on the inside as well. There is nothing healthy about replacing real food with fat-free products that look like real food, except for the absence of any nutritional benefit!

When Somersizing, you are eating delicious foods in combinations that make your digestive system run like clockwork. Food is digested quickly and efficiently. Your body extracts what it needs and discards the remainder while you melt away pounds and have more energy than ever before. And because it's so easy to eat this way, you can easily dine in just about any restaurant, and you can prepare meals for yourself by using any of my Somersize recipes or creating Somersize favorites of your own. Simple. Effective. Incredible!

Later on when you reach your goal weight, you will graduate to Level Two, the maintenance portion of the program. We loosen the reins a bit and show you how to Somersize for the rest of your life, without your weight fluctuating more than a couple of pounds.

That's the basic overview of the program. Those of you who did not read my first book, *Eat Great, Lose Weight,* are probably still skeptical. I understand. We have been so brainwashed into thinking a low-fat, low-calorie diet is the only way to safely lose weight that any program contrary to that notion sounds like quackery. I promise I will not lead you astray. I have always believed that my program is safe and effective because I garnered information from many doctors and nutritionists while creating it. But this information is on the cutting edge and not universally accepted. Now, because of Dr. Schwarzbein's additional clinical research on sugar and fat, I have the science to back it up. Not only is Somersizing safe and effective, it is *essential* to our health.

Sugar—The Real Culprit

One of the most important aspects of Somersizing is the elimination of sugar and foods high in starch (white flour, white rice, potatoes, and the like) that immediately turn to sugar upon digestion. I was shocked when I heard that the average American eats over 150 pounds of sugar and sweeteners (like corn syrup) every year! That's up 28 pounds since the early 1970s! We start off our morning with sugary cereals, Pop-Tarts, or a Danish. Or we look for low-fat, supposedly healthy alternatives like Nutri-Grain bars, granola, and muffins. A muffin is cake in a single serving size! These products are still loaded with sugar and often plenty of chemicals and preservatives.

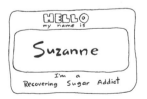

I understand the addiction to sugar as well as anyone because I am a recovering sugar addict. My body used to crave sweets, especially an hour or two after a meal. When you work in television there is always a large table covered with snacks called the "craft service" table. Around two in the afternoon I would find myself hovering around the table, maybe popping a little piece of chocolate into my mouth or a freshly baked cookie . . . and maybe just a corner of that brownie. I knew I was being naughty by snacking on junk food, but I thought the fat was the problem. I never linked my dips in energy to my sugar intake. I never knew my sugar intake was responsible for my irritability. I never knew my sugar intake was responsible for my rolling hips. And I never knew that eating sugar made me crave more and more sugar. Then I finally learned that *sugar is the body's greatest enemy!* Surprisingly, sugar is more fattening than fat.

Sugars and starches are carbohydrates. Carbohydrates are one of the body's main sources of fuel. The other is fat. In order to understand why some carbohydrates can cause weight problems, let's look at what happens when you eat carbos. When you eat carbos, they break down into glucose, which causes your blood sugar to rise. When the blood sugar is elevated, it is the job of the pancreas to secrete a hormone called insulin. Insulin balances the blood sugar by carrying the glucose to the cells, where it will be burned off for energy. By storing the sugar in the cells, your body balances your blood sugar level.

If we continue to eat too many carbohydrates at one time, insulin levels get higher and higher, and the cells need less and less energy. Most sugar is then stored as fat, and our energy-burning cells become resistant to the action of insulin or what is termed "insulin resistant." When the blood sugar is not accepted into the cells to be burned as fuel, it will be converted into fat, where it will be stored for later use. This explains how even fat-free carbohydrates, like sugar and white flour, can be converted to fat if we do not need the energy at the time we eat. In summary, eating too many carbohydrates at one time raises our blood sugar, causing the hormone insulin to be elevated. If the insulin cannot be balanced, due to insulin resistance, our entire hormonal system can become imbalanced, and hormonal imbalance leads to weight gain.

Most of us will experience some degree of insulin resistance because it occurs naturally as we get older (explaining why many of us gain weight as we age). Quite simply, as

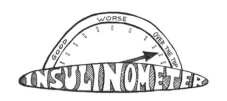

we get older our metabolic processes slow down and we do not need as many carbohydrates as we did when we were young. But if we don't change our eating habits, those carbohydrates we used to burn off as energy start to get converted to fat, and we get thick around the middle as the decades stack up.

Many of us have varying degrees of insulin resistance leading to weight gain and disease. Even some children have a genetic predisposition to insulin resistance. That's why the crux of this program is to teach you how to keep your pancreas from oversecreting insulin, which will keep your blood sugar balanced. The result is healing your insulin resistance so that the carbohydrates you do eat will be burned as fuel rather than stored as fat.

The amount your blood sugar is elevated depends upon the amount and the *type* of carbohydrates you are eating. Carbohydrates in their refined form are much harder on our systems than those in their natural form. In the last century we have refined most of the nutrients out of our foods. Whoever decided that rice would be better without the nutty brown shell? Brown rice has a wonderful flavor and is loaded with fiber you won't find in white rice. And how about white flour? Breads and pastas used to be made with natural whole grains, and as the grains became more refined, we as a society gained more and more weight.

Some studies show that 75 percent of the average American diet is made up of refined carbohydrates like sugar, white flour, white pasta, and instant potatoes. It's no wonder that obesity is epidemic in our country! And being thin is not just a vanity issue. It is a cause for great concern regarding your health. Obesity is the number two cause of premature death next to cigarette smoking.

Here's why this consumption of so many refined carbohydrates is hard on our system. Complex carbohydrates (like whole grains and vegetables low in starch) cause moderate to minimal increases in your blood sugar. But simple carbohydrates (like sugar, white flour, and potatoes) cause a sharp increase in blood sugar. This surge of blood sugar gives us a "sugar rush" or a "sugar high." As we now know, when the blood sugar is elevated to such a high level, insulin tries to store the sugar in the cells, but if they become filled with sugar, they will not accept any more. Then the pancreas secretes even more insulin to attempt to balance the blood sugar. This results in an excess amount of insulin in the bloodstream, which causes a condition called "hyperinsulinemia." The higher the insulin levels, the more sugar is converted and stored as fat. (One of the leading theories is that type II diabetes occurs when the fat cells are also filled, which means the sugar has *nowhere* to go and remains in the bloodstream.)

It makes me crazy when I see companies promoting fat-free items loaded with sugar and carbohydrates that will make your insulin levels go through the roof. And the chemicals that accompany many fat-free products are harmful to your health. Oles-tra, the fake fat recently approved by the FDA, must carry a warning label because it binds to some vitamins and nutrients so that they cannot be absorbed by your body. And it may cause abdominal cramping and loose stool syndrome. Is it really worth it for a bag of fat-free Lay's Wow! potato chips? Yes, you might say, "Wow!" after you eat the chips: "Wow! I wish I had an extra pair of panties in my purse." Besides, it's not the fat in the potato chips that makes you gain weight . . . it's the potato that raises insulin. Fat causes virtually no insulin response. Effective marketing has duped our society into thinking if we are eating low-fat, we are safely eating food that is healthier for us and will not make us fat. But they don't tell you that *fake food is harmful to your health* and *sugar turns right to fat!*

After extra insulin has sent the sugar to the fat cells, eventually our blood sugar is lowered to even below its starting point. That's when we feel the let-down or the "sugar low." This sugar low leaves us feeling tired, listless, and artificially hungry. During this time we often feel like taking a nap, or we reach for something sweet or caffeinated to give us more energy—then the vicious cycle repeats. Sugar goes in, blood sugar goes up, pancreas secretes insulin, then blood sugar drops and we feel tired and hungry again, causing us to eat more and more without ever satisfying our nutritional needs.

Now you are beginning to see the importance of insulin in determining whether the broken-down sugar will be burned as fuel or stored as fat. As I mentioned, some complex carbos cause smaller insulin responses (whole grains, green vegetables) and can be utilized immediately by the cells as fuel. Other carbos cause larger insulin responses (sugar, white flour, potatoes) and will often be stored as fat because they contain way more energy than our bodies need for immediate use. One nutritionist told me that a single potato provides us with more carbohydrates than some people need in an entire day! Think about how many excess carbohydrates you eat in a normal day, and imagine how much your body actually needs for fuel and how much gets stored as fat. Unless you're a marathon runner, you're probably storing an ample supply of fat reserves from overindulging in the wrong kinds of carbohydrates.

Now I know what some of you are thinking: How come I have friends who live on tons of bad carbs like junk food, candy bars, cheeseburgers with French fries, and they are thin as rails? The answer is that each of us is created differently, with a unique and ever-changing metabolism. Some people have a metabolism that will always burn the food they eat as fuel rather than storing it as fat. Other people start out burning off all their food as fuel, and as they get older their metabolism changes and suddenly they find themselves with a weight problem. But nothing is free. Even if your skinny friends can burn extra energy, they still can be damaged by eating junk food. They may not gain weight, but they are prone to heart attacks, decreased energy, mood swings, and increased incidence of death from poor nutrition.

Whatever the case, Somersizing is the answer. By eliminating foods that cause large fluctuations in our blood sugar and by properly combining nutritious, delicious foods, we are able to lose weight and gain energy while achieving our maximum health. Most of us do not have a perfect metabolism, but Somersizing can show you how to *get control* over your metabolism. This program can actually heal your ailing metabolism. It's never too late to change.

YOUR BODY . . . A FAST-RUNNING, FAT-BURNING MACHINE!

When your body needs energy, it will first look for carbohydrates to burn as fuel. If there are fewer carbohydrate sources available, your body will break down your fat reserves when you need energy. By cutting back on sugar and highly starchy foods, you force your body to use your fat reserves as an energy source.

That's the key to Somersizing. We convert our bodies from carbo-burning machines into fat-burning machines. By limiting our sugars and starches, we force our bodies to break down our fat reserves to use as a constant source of energy. No sugar highs and lows—just an even source of energy to get through the day as we watch our fat melt away.

The good news is that you don't have to say good-bye to sugar and starches forever. While you are on the weight loss portion of the program, Level One, the built-up sugar is being emptied from your cells. When you reach your goal weight, you will advance to Level Two, the maintenance portion of Somersizing. In Level Two you may incor-

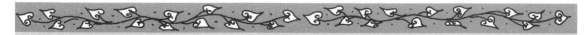

A SOMERSIZING SUCCESS STORY

Dear Suzanne,

Let me begin by thanking God for your book!

My husband and I slowly kept gaining weight, and before we realized, I had ballooned up to 190 pounds and Kevin was weighing in at 275 pounds. We looked, and more important, we felt bad. I have tried so many diets (all have portion control) and, yes, I would lose weight; my husband would lose weight. As soon as we would start to eat again, we would gain it back and then some more.

We have twin boys (three years old); and at the time I had absolutely no energy to keep up with them. I bought your book and we decided to give it a try. I couldn't believe we could eat all of this food and lose weight. I told my husband this cannot work, but we will try it anyway. Well, two weeks later he lost 15 pounds and I was down 9 pounds.

We still could not believe this could work. But now, 15 months later, I am 70 pounds lighter and Kevin lost 80 pounds. This is a way of life for us now. It is truly a wonderful way of life!

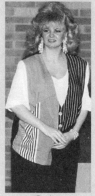

Before

I have to tell you we lost all this weight without exercising. Everybody wanted to know how we did it! When we told them, they bought the book!

Thank you so much for sharing this lifestyle with us!

God Bless,
Taylor and Kevin Kibodeaux

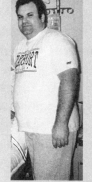

Before

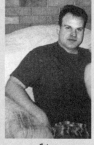

After

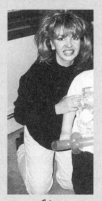

After

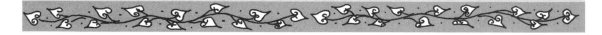

porate some sugar and starches back into your eating plans (in moderation). Because your cells are no longer filled with sugar, they can handle moderate amounts without becoming overloaded. On Level Two some previously forbidden sugars and starches are permitted because they will be burned off rather than stored as fat.

But what about eating fat? you ask. How can we change our metabolism if we're still eating fat? You'll be surprised at what you find in the next chapter.

THREE

Fat—The Fall Guy

In the last decade fat has been portrayed as the major villain leading to poor health and excess weight. We've all been watching our fat intake so we can lose that weight, right? Well, would it surprise you to know that in the last decade Americans have cut their fat intake from 38 percent to 34 percent of their daily calories, yet in that same time period the average weight per person has increased by eight pounds! How can that be? Isn't a reduced-fat diet supposed to help us lose weight? Doesn't less fat in our diets mean less fat on our bodies?

Not necessarily. We keep hearing, "Eat less fat. Eat less fat," and we have obeyed. Why, then, has the percentage of adults who are overweight *increased* by 10 percent since 1980? Over 37 percent of females and 34 percent of males are now overweight. Obesity is rampant in our country, and fat has been made the fall guy.

One of the first things people challenge me on when they hear about Somersizing is the fat issue. When you Somersize, yes, you can eat cheese. Yes, you can eat a juicy steak with a mushroom cream sauce. Yes, you can eat chicken with lemon butter sauce. Yes, you can eat taco salad topped with salsa and sour cream. Yes, you can eat tuna salad or egg salad with real mayonnaise.

WHEN YOU SOMERSIZE, YOU CAN EAT FAT AND STILL LOSE WEIGHT

That's right. Putting fat in your mouth will not add fat to your thighs. Eating dietary fat causes virtually no secretion of insulin, and as we learned in the last chapter, insulin must be present to store fat in the fat cells. Regardless of how much fat you eat, the pancreas will not secrete insulin, *which is the only way fat can be stored as body fat.* As long as you are combining properly, you can eat fat and still lose weight. But you can gain weight if you eat proteins or fats *with* carbohydrates. The combination of bread with cheese can be a killer. Here's why.

If you eat a Protein/Fat alone, like a piece of cheese, your body will break it down easily. And Pro/Fats will not cause weight gain when eaten alone because they trigger virtually no increase in your blood sugar levels, so there is not a significant insulin response. Pro/Fats can also be eaten in combination with vegetables low in starch (which are also foods that cause little to no insulin production). Therefore, eating Pro/Fats will not make you fat when eaten in the suggested Somersize combinations.

But let's say you eat fat *with* a carbohydrate, like cheese with white bread. The body *should* use the carbohydrates in the bread and the fat in the cheese for energy. But the carbohydrates in the bread will trigger an insulin response that can lead to both the bread *and* the cheese being sent to the fat cells to be stored as fat instead. So say good-bye to grilled-cheese sandwiches on white bread!

Believe it or not, fat is not fattening when eaten alone. You can eat fat with other fats, with proteins, or with vegetables in Somersize combinations and still lose weight. And what a pleasure it is to eat this way! I have never felt so indulged on a weight loss program.

Please don't misunderstand; I'm not suggesting you go out and gorge on fat. I still choose lean meats, and I prefer olive oil to butter. But I joyfully treat myself to cheese soufflé, butter sauce, or a piece of Brie without guilt. How wonderful not to feel deprived when you're trying to lose weight! I think that's the main reason Somersizing has been so successful with everyone who has tried it. You can incorporate rich, flavorful foods into your diet and still lose all the weight you want; and that helps people stick to the program.

FAT—FRIEND OR FOE?

Sometimes in life we stumble upon paths without even realizing it. As I said, after my last book, *Eat Great, Lose Weight,* I was challenged to death on the fat and cholesterol issue by everyone, from friends to co-workers to talk show hosts. "Okay," they would say, "so maybe you can eat fat and still lose weight, but what about increased cholesterol, the risk of heart disease, and certain types of cancer?"

I knew from my previous research that most of those ills were blamed on dietary fat, when actually insulin resistance was responsible for many of the maladies of modern day. (Later in this book you can read about the numerous studies that back up these claims.) Eating in proper Somersize combinations lowers insulin levels, which subsequently helps lower your cholesterol, and I've heard it time and time again from all of you who have seen the results for yourself.

Since my recent introduction to Dr. Diana Schwarzbein, I now have even more information based on her clinical findings, which corroborate not only that fat is not dangerous to our health . . . it is essential to

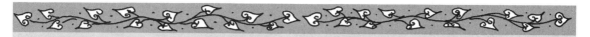

Dear Suzanne,

I have had a history of high cholesterol. Before medication (two different kinds), it was 514; after medicine it came down to 315. I watched the fat using canola oil and nonfat products, but my weight stayed up; and if the HDL got better, the LDL got worse; so it was a balancing act.

Since I bought your book I've lost 30 pounds in 5 months! Recently I went in for a blood test to check my cholesterol. My test amazed my doctor because in those months it had gone down from 315 to 225, the lowest he had ever seen in my medical history. He asked what I had done. I told him about your food plan.

I still want to lose at least 20 more pounds. I'm 69 and have been on all different kinds of diets through the years. Yours works. Keep up the good work.

Sincerely,
Jacque Slater

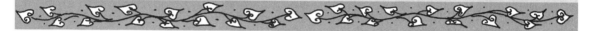

our health! I enthusiastically want to share this information! Dr. Schwarzbein explains in her book, *The Schwarzbein Principle,* the important role of fat in creating healthy cells. If we do not eat enough dietary fat, we are damaging our cells and our bodies' ability to reproduce new cells. When cell abnormalities develop, disease sets in.

Dr. Schwarzbein explains that a balanced diet, including fat, is essential to life. Now when I say fat, I don't mean the fat you give your body in the form of French fries or fat from a candy bar. Recently I was having lunch with a friend, and she ordered the typical low-fat dieter's lunch. I was sharing this information about fat with her, and by the end of the meal she was ordering a piece of cake and kidding, "I have to get my fat!" Please don't misunderstand. Don't use fat as

an excuse to eat junk food. The health benefit comes from eating *real* fat in its natural state, like butter, oil, cheese, sour cream, or fat found in meat or fish. Real fat is necessary to make hormones, and hormones are essential for breaking down old cells and making new ones. We must have sufficient hormones to make healthy cells, and we must have healthy cells to make more hormones.

Dr. Schwarzbein goes on to further explain that in the normal aging process hormone levels will decline, causing the subsequent loss of healthy cells. Simply, aging results when our bodies break down more cells than they build up. Although there is no way to prevent *normal* metabolic aging, our society is on a frightening path toward what Dr. Schwarzbein calls "accelerated metabolic aging." Bad eating habits, stress, caffeine, alcohol abuse, and inactivity can lead to extended periods of high-insulin levels that prematurely age our bodies on a cellular level. This aging process leads to disease.

Dr. Schwarzbein warns that when the hormone insulin is present at increased levels, it can disrupt every other hormone system in the body, which can lead not only to excessive body fat, but to degenerative diseases of aging such as different types of cancer, cholesterol abnormalities, coronary artery disease, high blood pressure, osteoporosis, stroke, and type II diabetes. *Hormone imbalances always lead to disease.* We must control our insulin levels so as not to disrupt every other hormone system in the body! For instance, Dr. Schwarzbein explains that high insulin levels in women lead to increased testosterone levels, which blunt the effects of estrogen in the body, which can lead to no ovulation and decreased production of the sex hormone progesterone. Therefore, poor eating habits can actually send women into early menopause . . . all from eating the wrong kinds of carbohydrates!

Furthermore, Dr. Schwarzbein says, women who are already going through menopause are at extreme risk of disease. As women age, we naturally become more insulin resistant, which explains why it gets harder to stay slim as we get older. Adopting a high-carb diet exacerbates the problem because all those carbohydrates increase insulin resistance. As I said earlier, the elevated amount of insulin in the blood can increase testosterone levels, which further blunts the production of the female sex hormones estrogen and progesterone. Compound the problem with a low-fat diet and you have even less hormone production (because we must consume dietary fat to create hormones). Besides the uncomfortable side effects of hot flashes, cramping, and mood swings, an imbalance of these sex hormones means we cannot produce healthy cells. As Dr. Schwarzbein has helped me learn, it is at this critical stage that women become vulnerable to disease. If hormones are not present to rebuild healthy cells, the cells become damaged. These abnormal cells invite disease. We must eat fat in order to create hormones to keep our cells healthy. (In addition to a balanced diet, including protein, fat, fruit, whole grains, and vegetables, make sure to discuss hormone replacement with your doctor if you are going through menopause. Synthetic hormones such as Premarin or Provera simply remove the *symptoms* of menopause, whereas natural hormones actually replace lost hormones.)

This information is astounding to me! I have always understood the connection between nutrition and health, but never has it been so clear. Everything we put into our mouths, good or bad, has a direct effect on our health. We all know eating junk food is bad for us, yet I don't think we consider the consequences of the bad food choices we make. Years of poor eating habits cumulatively add up to damaged cells and our bodies' inability to produce new, healthy cells. When we eat poorly we age faster, not only externally, but internally as well. And this accelerated metabolic aging process leaves us vulnerable to disease at an earlier age.

Processed foods also introduce free radicals into our systems. Free radicals are molecules that carry an extra electron. Since electrons need to be paired off, these free radicals roam through our system like little home wreckers, trying to steal electrons from healthy cells. This process damages our system on a cellular level. Antioxidants such as vitamin E, vitamin A, and vitamin C help to neutralize free radicals. When we replace real food (which includes natural vitamins) with processed food, we are not supplying our body with the natural antioxidants it needs to fight the free radicals; instead we are introducing more free radicals into our system! The damage that results over time accelerates the metabolic aging process and leads to insulin resistance, then disease and early death. Ironically, two of the most powerful antioxidants, vitamin A and vitamin E, are found in foods that contain fat.

Not only are we a nation that eats processed foods in abundance, consider that the average American also drinks forty-two gallons of sugary soft drinks every year! We are literally killing ourselves with sugar and chemicals that break down our bodies on a cellular level. The sugar and caffeine in one cola wreak havoc on your body by spiking insulin levels. Think about it every time you consider having a can of soda. Imagine the insulin in your body looking unsuccessfully for places to store the abundance of glucose and visualize how the sugar then gets converted into fat because your cells just cannot accept any more sugar.

With diet drinks you don't have the sugar to contend with, but you have the additional free radicals from the artificial sweeteners. To help you stop drinking diet drinks, let me share with you the most recent studies on the frightening effects of aspartame. Lab studies have proven irreversible brain damage in laboratory animals. In fact, one can of soda can raise the levels of toxins in the brain of an infant higher than levels that caused brain damage in immature animals. Certainly no one is filling infants' bottles with diet sodas, but many toddlers and children drink this poison regularly. And thousands of adults drink diet sodas by the gallon. Since there are not yet any long-term studies showing the effects of aspartame, is it really worth the risk? All for a can of diet cola? I think not.

The overall picture has never been so clear to me. I visualize all my happy little cells. As I get older I know some of them will die off, and there is nothing I can do about that. But I imagine what happens when I am not giving my body the proper combination of nutritious foods, and I see the cells dying off at a rapid rate. But when I give my body the protein, fat, and complex carbohydrates it needs, my cells thrive and I feel empowered that I can stave off disease and aging for as long as possible. How wonderful to realize that Somersizing not only keeps me in control of my weight, but keeps me at my metabolic prime. I know the food I am eating is creating millions of happy cells that keep me young, slim, and healthy.

FOUR

Dangers of a Low-Fat, High-Carb Diet

Now that we understand the importance of eating fat as well as the dangers of eating too much sugar and starch, let's explore the well-known food pyramid recommended by the United States Department of Agriculture. The USDA recommends our daily breakdown of foods to include 60 percent carbohydrates, with 15 percent protein and no more than 25 percent fat. Following this food plan will only make your body appear the same shape as the pyramid! All those carbohydrates are responsible for sending that insulin through the roof, which packs on the pounds and creates all those other physical ailments resulting from raised insulin. Carbohydrates are mostly used by our bodies only as a fuel source, and since our bodies can create our own fuel source from our fat reserves, or from protein and fats, carbohydrates are not considered an essential part of our meal plans. Fat and protein, on the other hand, create virtually no

rise in insulin levels and provide our bodies with the building materials needed for good health. Therefore Somersizing recommends you turn the pyramid upside down, eating mostly protein, fats, and vegetables, with minimal amounts of carbohydrates. And when you do . . . watch your figure change shape, just like the turned-over pyramid!

We've been so trained to think that a diet low in fat is the *only* way to lose weight. But I'm telling you that a low-fat diet does not guarantee you will lose weight. What you

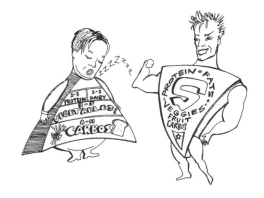

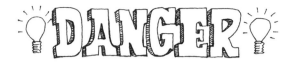

are eating *in place of* that fat will have a lot to do with determining how much weight you lose. Fat-free pastries, fat-free cookies, fat-free cakes, low-fat potato chips, reduced-fat crackers, fat-free caramel rice cakes, fat-free licorice, nonfat frozen yogurt . . . less fat? Yes. Lose weight? No way.

Junk food is junk food, whether it's fat-free or not. It's nearly impossible to lose weight if you're filling up on these so-called healthy snack alternatives. Most of these products are empty foods that leave your body nutritionally unsatisfied and hungry for a decent meal. And of course by now you know the culprit in all of these fat-free products . . . *sugar!* I'll say it again . . . *sugar is more fattening than fat.* Besides the sugar, these products often have white flour and a host of chemicals that your body does not need or appreciate. I have a friend who used to eat a large nonfat frozen yogurt every day. She figured it was basically a "free food" since it was low in calories and had no fat. She couldn't figure out why she was gaining weight. I explained that it was the sugar.

Sugar is the body's greatest enemy; and don't forget, *fat is your friend.* Let me further explain why a low-fat diet can be dangerous to your health. We must eat protein and fat to make hormones that regulate the systems of the body and promote healthy cells. Proteins and fat are necessary for the constant rebuilding that takes place in our bodies. When we do not supply our bodies with

these essential nutrients, as Dr. Schwarzbein explains, our bodies will break down our *muscles* and *bones* to derive the materials they need for rebuilding.

Although the scale may say you are losing weight on a low-fat, high-carbohydrate diet, you are actually losing more muscle and bone mass than you are fat. But, again, your body will kick into survival mode and slow down your metabolic processes to halt the depletion of your bones and muscle mass. It is at this point that you experience the tired feelings that accompany low-fat, high-carb diets. Low-fat diets deprive our bodies of protein and fat, the essential elements we need for living. Although you may decrease your bodily fat initially, you will also decrease your lean muscle mass. When you go off the low-fat diet and resume your normal eating habits, you will gain back more fat than before.

Plus, muscle mass is necessary for helping to decrease insulin levels. Muscle provides another area for insulin to stow away elevated blood sugar, so that it does not get converted to fat. If we deplete our lean muscle mass, insulin has fewer places to store sugar. This leads to insulin resistance, which we know is the reason we pack on the extra pounds.

The midsection is the first area where insulin tends to store fat. It makes sense that as we age normally we get a spare tire around the middle, since we naturally become more insulin resistant. And if we are on an "accelerated metabolic aging" path, we are becoming insulin resistant at an even earlier age, which will lead not only to weight gain, but to disease. Body beware the deadly spare tire around the midsection—it is a sure sign of elevated insulin levels!

Somersizing encourages appropriate proteins, fats, vegetables low in starch, and fruit in proper combinations to unload the built-up sugar in our system. This unloading is the burning of fat stores. As our system unloads, we lower our insulin resistance and begin to reprogram our metabolism. In addition, because we are giving our bodies essential nutrients, we are decreasing excess body fat while building lean muscle mass. And by regulating the hormonal systems of the body, we can discover the key to preventing disease. How wonderful that eating delicious, flavorful, nutritious foods will help keep our insulin levels stabilized, so we can lose weight and slow down the aging process.

CHOLESTEROL AND HEART DISEASE—THE REAL TRUTH

If you have high cholesterol, you've probably been hounded by your doctors and your family members to cut back on foods high in fat and cholesterol. But is your low-fat diet helping to lower your cholesterol? Doubtful. Only 20 percent of the cholesterol found in your blood is a direct result of the foods you eat. The remaining amount is produced by your liver from excess sugars (carbohydrates). Although it seems logical that cutting back on fatty foods will decrease your total cholesterol levels, in actuality the less fat you eat, the higher the rate of cholesterol production in the liver.

Though this is contrary to what most people think, as I learned from Dr. Schwarzbein, cholesterol and fat are absolutely *essential* to good health. They are used by the body as building materials and are in need of constant replenishment from the foods we eat. Cholesterol is used to make important hormones such as estrogen, testosterone, progesterone, DHEA, and the antistress hormone cortisol. When we deprive our bodies of cholesterol, the compound the body uses to make these hormones, cell membrane structure is altered and cell growth is disrupted. This causes an increased risk of cancer because cancer arises from the abnormal division of cells. In addition, a lack of cholesterol in our diets can lead to depression and irritability.

It took some time for me to finally accept this information, but after spending time with Dr. Schwarzbein I realize how important it is to understand the connection between cholesterol and carbohydrates. Spread the word . . . we must include cholesterol in our diets to stay healthy. If we do not eat cholesterol, our body will produce its own cholesterol by converting the carbohydrates we eat into cholesterol. Again, insulin plays an important role in the cholesterol equation. Insulin activates an enzyme in your liver called HMG Co-A Reductase, which causes your liver to overproduce cholesterol from the carbohydrates you eat. When insulin levels are high, the liver produces more cholesterol. It is this internal overproduction of cholesterol that contributes to the formation of damaging artery plaque that can lead to heart attack and stroke.

Dear Suzanne,

I have lost 51 pounds and 45 inches in 10 months. I lost 20 pounds and 18³/₄ inches in the first two months! I have an underactive thyroid and polycystic ovaries, both of which tend to cause added weight, and I am a carbohydrate lover. I never understood why I had gained so much weight since I never ate a lot of fat, but I did eat a lot of carbohydrates. Your book made it so easy to understand how the digestive process works and how carbohydrates turn into stored fat.

I had lost 50 pounds about six years ago, but I had to severely limit my calories—below 1000 per day, which I now know is bad for you. Of course, as soon as I went back to eating normally, my weight came back on. It was very discouraging and depressing.

With Somersizing I don't count calories or measure portions. I feel so much healthier and I know I *am* healthier. I do not crave sugar at all; in fact the few times that I have eaten desserts I don't really like them because they taste too sweet. The recipes are delicious, easy to follow, and don't require hard-to-find ingredients.

As you always say "this is not a diet, it is a way of life." I can easily see myself Somersizing forever. Why wouldn't I—I've lost more than ¹/₄ of my total body weight, I get tons of compliments, I am healthier, and I feel more energetic. Who can argue with those benefits!

Thank you so much for your inspiration and help.

Sincerely,
Debbie Thomas

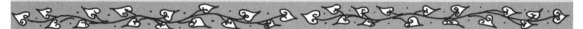

Finally, this information makes such sense to me! Especially in how it relates to my family. My husband, Alan, is a fruitaholic. He loves fruit. I remember one summer we were planning a trip to Majorca, Spain. Alan had heard about the amazing Valencia oranges from the region and was looking forward to tasting them. When we got to the island, we spent days driving around looking for these oranges, but they were not to be found. Soon the entire vacation became about looking for fruit. It was like being with a drug addict going through withdrawal; he had to have his fruit fix!

When we finally found some fruit, it wasn't even very good, but Alan ate it anyway to temper his craving.

In fact, for years Alan would skip lunch or dinner and opt to eat all fruit. He fancied himself the picture of health. When he went to the doctor, however, he was told his cholesterol level was dangerously high—255. His doctors, as one would expect, told him to cut back on foods high in cholesterol and fat. He explained that his diet was already low in fat and that he ate mostly fruits and vegetables. They told him to cut back the fat and cholesterol even more.

Fearing for his health, Alan cut out virtually all the eggs, meat, and cheese that he used to enjoy in moderation in his regular diet. He cut back on the butter and cream and ate, guess what . . . more fruit! In addition, he ate fresh vegetables and plenty of pasta.

Before too long I started to notice that Alan was getting a little paunchy around the middle. I told him all that fruit must be making him fat. He laughed. "Fruit doesn't make you fat," he'd say. "Besides, I have to watch my cholesterol." Surprisingly, when Alan went back to the doctor to have his cholesterol level checked, it had actually gone from 255 to 265! How could that be? He was eating little to no cholesterol and fat, yet his cholesterol had actually increased. The doctors were baffled and decided to put him on pills to lower his cholesterol.

Now it makes such sense to me! Alan's insulin levels were through the roof from the excessive amount of fruit and carbohydrates he was consuming. Alan was a victim of elevated insulin levels, which were causing weight gain (because the sugar was being converted to fat) and increased cholesterol (because he wasn't eating the necessary cholesterol his body needed, the enzyme in his liver caused his liver to convert the carbohydrates he was eating into cholesterol). The key to lowering Alan's cholesterol levels was to eat less fruit and pasta and to eat *more* foods with cholesterol and fat. And it worked. He is now off the medication and eating a more balanced diet, including moderate amounts of fruit, protein, fat, and complex carbohydrates, in proper combinations to keep his blood sugar levels balanced. Without the high insulin levels surging through his bloodstream, I'm happy to report that once again he's thin around the middle and his cholesterol level is now down to an amazing 178!

When you Somersize, you are encouraged to eat real foods that help increase your HDL, the good cholesterol in your bloodstream. This good cholesterol is responsible for fighting off heart disease. Eating a diet too low in fat has been shown to lower your HDL. That's why when you Somersize, I encourage you to eat foods that increase your HDL, like olive oil, butter, and fish oil, and foods that help decrease your overall cholesterol, like lean meats, fresh fish, and unsaturated oils. Most important, you are controlling your insulin levels, which is the key to controlling cholesterol levels.

So that's the skinny on fat and cholesterol. Make sure to include it in your meals by eating proteins/fats with vegetables and you will not gain weight or increase your cholesterol. In fact, you will lose weight because you will change your metabolism so your body uses more and more energy, thus forcing your system to burn your fat reserves. Plus you will lower your cholesterol by giving your body the essential cholesterol and fat it needs to thrive.

FIVE

Pick the Healthy Option

These days it's hard to know what to believe when you are trying to choose the best way to lead a healthy life. The same cycles seem to repeat over and over. It starts with the medical community publishing a study. Then the media gets hold of the information and barrages us with warnings. Then the manufacturers play off our fears and produce products designed to promote "health."

For example, in the seventies it was salt. A medical study showed a relationship between salt consumption and high blood pressure. Then the media got hold of the information and put all their efforts into scaring us to death about the effects of salt. Suddenly everyone was worrying about too much salt causing water retention and heart attacks. And the manufacturers followed suit by putting big labels on their products: "LOW IN SODIUM." We became obsessed with counting our sodium grams.

"Watch out for pickles and pretzels—they've got enough salt for an entire week."

Then the salt scare became old news, and the morning shows needed a new topic for their "health" segment. Suddenly there was a new medical study, a new media frenzy, and the birth of a new demon . . . fat. Everyone started counting fat grams to keep slim and ward off heart attacks. Don't eat that chicken skin. Hold the sour cream. Cheese is the enemy. Then came the manufacturers and their products. It's gotta be nonfat to be good for you. "Bring on the pickles and the pretzels . . . they're fat-free." And we continue to buy it all. "Hey, look, chocolate syrup has no fat . . . bring it on."

I know what you're thinking: Now it's sugar. All of a sudden you're being told you need to be concerned with sugar over all else because sugar is the *real* reason we are overweight and unhealthy. It's confusing, and you are probably thinking, What am I supposed to believe? First we hear don't eat fat, now we hear you *must* eat fat and not eat sugar. But the warning about sugar is not a trend, and this weight loss program is not a fad. The effects of high insulin levels (resulting from overeating sugar/carbohydrates/caffeine or from stress) and their relationship to weight gain, abnormal cholesterol levels, coronary heart disease, and type II diabetes have been documented in numerous medical studies. I have listed several in the bibliography. This is hardly new information.

Specifically I want to share three articles, brought to my attention by Dr. Schwarzbein, linking high insulin levels to these diseases. The first is from the *New England Journal of Medicine,* which concluded that healthy persons with hyperinsulinemia and normal glucose levels are at higher risk for coronary artery disease, as compared with a well-matched group of healthy subjects with normal insulin levels. The second article is from *Diabetes Care.* I'll share with you a passage from the summary:

> . . . much evidence has begun to accumulate that chronic day-long hyperinsulinemia is associated with the development of hypertension [high blood pressure], hyperlipidemia [high cholesterol and triglycerides], and atherosclerosis [clogged arteries]. In a sense, insulin resistance can be viewed as a large iceberg submerged just below the surface of the water. The physician recognizes only the tip of the iceberg—diabetes, obesity, hypertension, hypertriglyceridemia, diminished HDL-chol, and atherosclerosis—which extrude above the surface, and complete insulin

resistance may be missed. The medical community is treating only the *symptoms* of insulin resistance, rather than attacking the root of the problem, which is the insulin resistance itself.

The third article from *Diabetes Care* outlines the research on the subject of insulin for the last twenty years. This comprehensive study concludes: "The fact that hyperinsulinemia has been shown to have an independent predictive correlation with cardiovascular disease and that insulin has biological actions on arterial tissue, lipid metabolism, and renal sodium handling suggest that the primary abnormality may be hyperinsulinemia due to insulin resistance. . . ." Check out these articles for yourself to get the full story on how dangerous insulin resistance can be.

In contrast, there are *no* long-term studies regarding the negative effects of fat. In fact, Dr. Schwarzbein explained to me how the entire "fat scare" probably resulted from one lone study in 1981. A five-year study followed approximately 1,200 men who were healthy but considered high risk for coronary heart disease because they smoked and had high cholesterol levels. Half of the men were placed in the intervention group and instructed to stop smoking, eat less sugar, drink less alcohol, and reduce their cholesterol intake. The other half in the control group were to continue eating, drinking, and smoking as they always had.

The intervention group had checkups every six months and were encouraged to continue a healthier lifestyle, including reduced smoking and drinking. The control group had a checkup only once a year. At the end of the five-year study, those who had reduced their smoking, drinking, and cholesterol intake had decreased their heart disease and death by 47 percent over those who did not.

The results were certainly dramatic and made a serious impression on the medical community. These results, however, were grossly misinterpreted. The intervention group's lower cholesterol levels were attributed solely to eating less cholesterol (meat, eggs, butter, and the like), so the "fat-free" movement began. But what the study didn't document was the *insulin* levels in the intervention group as opposed to the control group's. The intervention group's decrease in sugar, alcohol, and smoking was not even considered a contributing effect in lowering cholesterol levels! And we know anything that lowers your insulin levels will create multiple benefits, including weight loss, lower cholesterol levels, and decreased risk of heart disease. What the intervention group *actually* showed was that smoking less, drinking less alcohol, and eating less sugar lowered insulin levels. And these lower insulin levels decreased cholesterol.

Because of this study, and the misinterpreted results, we've all been taught for the last two decades that eating less fat and cholesterol will help lower cholesterol levels. One study has changed the opinion about what connotes "healthy" eating. And remember, there are *no* long-term studies proving the negative effects of fat. All the hoopla in the fat-free movement is based on short-term studies. Meanwhile, as a society we've replaced dinners revolving around some kind of protein with meals made up predominantly of carbohydrates. To be more "healthy" we've replaced steak dinners with pasta dinners and pork chops with fried rice. Everything has become low-fat, but even though we've cut our fat intake in the last two decades, we've gained weight, increased our cholesterol, and heightened the incidence of cancer. The low-fat movement is not working! Carbohydrates are fuel for your body, but think about your car . . . it needs gas for fuel, but imagine how your engine would falter if you never gave it any oil! Your body needs "oil," too, which is why you must include fats and protein in your diet—to keep your engine running smoothly.

I hope, after reading this far, you have come to realize that fat is not your enemy. Coming off the "fat scare" decade, we need to reprogram ourselves about what constitutes the healthy option when deciding what to eat. I went to the market and picked up a few items, comparing full-fat products to fat-free products. Take a look at the difference in the ingredient lists of various mayonnaises:

MY HOMEMADE MAYONNAISE (FROM *EAT GREAT, LOSE WEIGHT*)

vegetable oil	salt
eggs	white pepper
vinegar	Tabasco
lemon juice	Worcestershire sauce

Calories per tablespoon: 100
Fat grams: 11 g

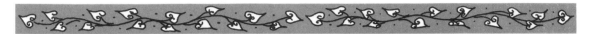

A SOMERSIZING SUCCESS STORY

Dear Suzanne,

I read your book as soon as I received it, made a menu plan then let it sit for a month before I started. If only I could get that month back! As you've said many times, "THE WEIGHT JUST FELL OFF!"

While on vacation from June 17 thru August, I LOST 27 POUNDS! I'm not a size 22 anymore; I'm a size 16 and still losing weight.

My blood pressure went from 151/98 to 124/77. My doctor praised my success during my checkup. She took me off both of my blood pressure medications and gave me a home monitor to use as I continue "Somersizing."

I will eat like this always! I work around food all day and know I will not gain weight again. Three of my co-workers took your book home after asking how I lost the weight.

I don't sit home like before. Going out and to dinner while wearing stylish clothes adds years to my life. This is the BEST, EASIEST, NO BRAINER way to eat and live life. Thank you!

Toni Chamberlain

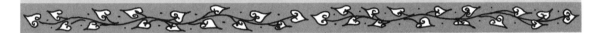

BEST FOODS MAYONNAISE

soybean oil
whole eggs
vinegar
water
egg yolks
salt
sugar
lemon juice
natural flavors
calcium disodium
    EDTA used to
    protect quality

Calories per tablespoon: 100
Fat grams: 11 g

BEST FOODS LOW FAT MAYONNAISE DRESSING

water
corn syrup
soybean oil
modified food starch
egg whites
vinegar
salt
maltodextrin
gums (cellulose gel
    and gum)
xanthan
carrageenan

natural flavors
color added
mustard flour
sodium benzoate
calcium disodium
    EDTA used to
    protect quality

Calories per tablespoon: 25
Fat grams: 1 g

KRAFT MIRACLE WHIP NONFAT DRESSING

water
sugar
natural and
    artificial flavor
    (contains egg*)
modified food
    starch
vinegar
contains less
    than 2% of
    cellulose gel
salt
citric acid
xanthan gum
dried cream*
artificial color

lactic acid
with potassium sorbate and calcium
   disodium EDTA as preservatives
yellow 6
phylloquinone (vitamin K$_1$)
Blue 1
trivial source of fat and cholesterol

Calories per tablespoon: 15
Fat grams: 0 g

Notice how much farther away we get from real food as we take the fat out of mayonnaise. The eggs and oil get replaced with sugar and starches. By the time you get to the fat-free Miracle Whip, you can hardly pronounce a single ingredient! Imagine what's happening to your body by ingesting a lifetime of chemicals and preservatives. How can anyone think that picking the fat-free product is the healthy option! We do, though, because we've been trained to look only at fat grams and calories. Yes, the low-fat and no-fat products are lower in fat and calories, but fat causes no insulin response and therefore will not be converted to fat. The sugars and starches, however, cause a rise in blood sugar, which triggers an insulin response, which can cause fat-free mayonnaise to be stored as fat.

Let's look at another example—ice cream:

BREYER'S NATURAL VANILLA

milk	sugar
cream	natural vanilla flavor

Calories per 1/2 cup: 150
Fat grams: 9 g
Carbohydrate: 15 g

DREYER'S FAT-FREE ICE CREAM

skim milk	mono and
sugar	diglycerides
corn syrup	tara gum
modified food	carrageenan
starch	dextrose
natural and artifi-	vitamin A
cial flavor	palmitate
cellulose gel	annatto color
cellulose gum	

Calories per 1/2 cup: 100
Fat grams: 0 g
Carbohydrate: 23 g

Again, look at the sugars, starches, and chemicals that take the place of real food when you extract the fat from ice cream. It's easy to think you're making a healthier choice by picking the fat-free item if you look only at the calories and fat. I wish these products had an insulin meter on the labels so we could see the effect on our blood sugar and the subsequent insulin levels. One reading that helps give some insight is the carbohydrate count. The real ice cream has 15 grams of carbohydrate per serving, while the fat-free product has 23 grams. The higher carbohydrate count means more insulin and all the negativity that goes with it. Plus, many people eat larger portions of fat-free products because they think there is no harm in eating something that is free of fat. If you're going to eat ice cream (on Level Two), please eat a moderate amount of *real* ice cream after a Pro/Fats meal for the least amount of imbalance.

Now let's analyze some breakfast meals to see the effect of sugars and fats.

Two eggs fried in butter (1 tablespoon)
Three pork sausage links
One sliced tomato

Calories: 425
Fat grams: 35 g
Carbohydrate: 1.5 g

A bowl of corn flakes (1 oz.)
Nonfat milk (8 oz.)
Banana
Glass of orange juice (6 oz.)

Calories: 381
Fat grams: <1 g
Carbohydrate: 84 g

Healthy Choice Low-fat Apple Spice
   Muffin
Glass of orange juice (6 oz.)

Calories: 280
Fat grams: 4 g
Carbohydrate: 66 g

If you were to place these breakfast options side by side and ask someone to rate them from the most healthy to the least healthy, they would probably rate the muffin or the cereal as the most, with the fried eggs and sausage as the least. But look at the carbohydrate content in the muffin breakfast: 66 grams. For many of us, that's more than we need for an entire day! Don't be fooled, folks. Muffins are an excuse to eat cake in the morning. Just because they contain apples, or bran, or are "low fat" doesn't mean they are healthy options. They are also loaded with sugar and white flour, which will send the insulin soaring.

Other people commonly mistake the cornflakes breakfast as a healthy option, because it is low in fat and cholesterol. But look at the carbohydrate count: 84 grams of carbohydrate will send insulin levels soaring.

I know it is hard to believe that eggs and sausages are a healthier choice than cereal with fresh fruit, juice, and nonfat milk. How can the breakfast highest in calories, fat, and cholesterol help us to lose weight and keep our bodies healthy? We must remember, excess calories and fat do not make us gain weight. *Hormonal imbalance leads to weight gain.* Insulin is a hormone, and when we eat foods that cause our insulin levels to rise, our entire hormonal system may become imbalanced, causing food to be stored as fat rather than burned as fuel. Even though the sausage-and-eggs meal is high in calories, fat, and cholesterol, eating it will cause little insulin response, leaving very little chance of this meal being stored as fat.

Plus, fat and cholesterol do not cause disease. In fact, they provide our bodies with the essential materials they need to rebuild and thrive. *Hormonal imbalance leads to disease.* Foods that create high insulin levels lead to hormonal imbalance, which can lead to disease and increased incidence of early death.

Reprogram your thinking by picking the healthy option and you'll be on your way to reprogramming your metabolism.

SIX

Food Combining—Fact or Fad?

Somersizing has helped over a million people to lose weight and gain vital energy while they heal their systems from years of bad food and lifestyle choices. But even after losing ten, twenty, thirty pounds, or more, many people still don't understand how a program with this much food and this much flavor can help you lose weight.

The theory behind food combining is that proteins and carbohydrates digest at different rates. Proteins require an acid environment to be digested, and carbohydrates require a base environment. When proteins and carbohydrates are eaten together, the enzymes cancel each other out, creating a halt in the digestion process. Many advocates support this theory, although there are challengers who argue that food combining is not based on scientific fact.

Here's what I know: Food combining works. Over a million of you have proven that to me, and frankly that's all the proof I

need! *Why* does it work? Although I am not a doctor or a nutritionist, I will try to explain how Somersizing works in the layman's terms I have come to understand. These are the facts that are scientifically proven when it comes to Somersizing:

When you eliminate sugar, white flour, and other funky foods, you force your body to burn off your fat reserves and use them as an energy source.

The elimination of sugar and foods high in starch, like potatoes and white rice, is the

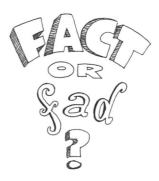

essential reason we lose weight on the Somersize system. Carbohydrates are one of the body's main sources of energy. Carbos are the fuel that keeps us going. But as we've learned, it is important to be eating the *right kinds* of carbohydrates. Whole grains, fruits, and vegetables low in starch are excellent sources of carbohydrates that give us energy and provide necessary fiber for proper elimination. But some carbohydrates, like sugar and foods very high in starch, are loaded with more energy than our bodies can use at a given time. This excess energy that isn't burned off will be stored as fat for later use. (Of course, your activity level determines that quotient.)

I cannot stress enough how crucial it is to understand that *sugar is more fattening than fat.* Even though sugars and starches are "fat-free," they have a tendency to turn right to fat. Think of a baked potato as one gigantic sugar cube and imagine the amount of excess energy you are giving your body! At first I grieved the loss of potatoes in my diet . . . after all, I was born Suzanne Mahoney, and I grew up on the Irish staple. But when I think not only about the potatoes, but about the *kinds* of carbos and the *amounts* of carbos I used to eat, I understand why I was gaining weight: toast or cereal in the morning, a sandwich for lunch, and pasta or meat with potatoes for dinner added up to way more energy than I needed to get through the day. All that extra sugar had no place to be stored in my cells, so it was converted to fat and stored away.

Sugar and foods high in starch can also put your blood sugar levels on a roller coaster that keeps you hungry and tired.

When you eat sugar or starch your blood sugar increases and you feel great. That's what we call the "sugar high." But before the blood sugar is leveled back to normal, it usually dips *below* its starting point. It is during this "sugar low" that we feel tired and often decide to reach for more sugar or caffeine to pick up our energy level. Well, watch the cycle repeat itself: we have a few cookies, and our blood sugar increases. At first we feel good, then our blood sugar decreases to below its starting point and we feel tired and hungry. Once again we reach for something sweet or caffeinated to keep our energy level up: in goes the candy bar, up goes the blood sugar, down goes the blood sugar, and so on and so on and so on. Sugars and certain starches are empty foods that cause highs and lows in our energy level, which in turn can cause us to eat way more than our actual appetites require.

When you Somersize, your energy level remains constant. You can eat as much as you want, but you will not overeat because you are giving your body good, nutritious foods that satisfy your appetite. It is not calories that lead to weight gain—it's imbalanced hormones. That is why you may eat until you are full . . . period.

Here's what I might eat in a typical day: fruit in the morning, followed by whole-grain toast or cereal; a hearty salad with grilled chicken and my choice of dressing for lunch; maybe a piece of cheese in the afternoon as a snack; and for dinner, chicken, meat, or fish with a lovely sauce, plenty of fresh, sautéed, steamed, or grilled vegetables, and a green salad with dressing of my choice. And guess what? Without

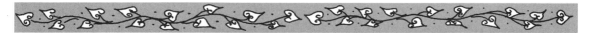

Dear Suzanne,

I am writing to thank you for your wonderful book *Eat Great, Lose Weight*. My story is a little different than most. I bought your book in October 1997 when I was about four months pregnant with my second child. About four years earlier, when I had my first child, I gained 50 pounds during that pregnancy and had a difficult time losing the weight. Finally, in 1996, I started to work out on a daily basis trying to get rid of the excess weight. Over the next year and a half I had worked off most of the weight I gained with pregnancy number one and started to work on the excess weight I had on my body before I got pregnant. Then, in June of 1997, I got pregnant again. My husband and I had such mixed emotions. We were happy because we always said we wanted four years' difference between our children and this was exactly what we were getting. Then we were both so sad because I was just starting to get trim and neither of us could bear the thought of me gaining 50 pounds again. To admit this to anyone else brings tears to my eyes, because it sounds so selfish to not be overwhelmed with joy about having another child, but we were both so caught up in my struggles with weight that it overshadowed our joy.

The first four months of my second pregnancy went along perfectly, as did my weight gain. I had gained about 14 pounds when a nurse practitioner counseled me on my eating habits. She said everything about my health was fine but my weight gain was slightly ahead of schedule. There I was, on my way to gaining 50 pounds (or more) again. Then I saw you on television explaining your program. It sounded easy enough and it made sense, so I told my husband about it and bought the book. Over the years I had tried most weight loss programs with limited success. I usually lost some weight at first; then, eventually, the weight would creep back on once I started to eat "real" food again. I had even been anorexic for about a year when I was 15 years old. During this time I was bone thin and learned the calorie content of every food known to man. I truly believe this is where I slowed down my metabolism to the point that I could not eat an average meal without gaining weight. My daily

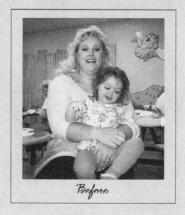

Before

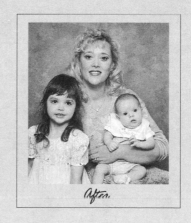

After

existence, during my entire adult life, consisted of always counting my calories and worrying about what I was eating or going to eat next.

When I got your book in October 1997, it took me about a week to get up the nerve to even open it because I was convinced that I was going to gain weight while I was pregnant. I felt helpless and your book didn't even inspire me at first. Then one Saturday afternoon I read it from cover to cover and decided to start eating the Somersize way the next day. The program was explained so well and was so simple to follow that it took me only about two weeks to have everything "memorized."

My results were astounding, to say the least. During the remainder of my pregnancy, I followed your program to the letter. I did not "cheat" at all and the weight fell off! Every month I went to the doctor's office and I would lose two to three pounds on the average. Now that might not sound like much, but everyone must remember that while I was shrinking, the baby was growing. My friends just could not believe their eyes. Some people even got angry with me because they were convinced that I was starving both the baby and myself. Nothing could have been further from the truth. I was actually eating more food than I ever had in my life; three full meals a day and at least two snacks a day. I basically ate whenever I got hungry and I ate until I was full. Another wonderful benefit of Somersizing was that I never got heartburn, which I was plagued with during the first pregnancy. I actually lost so much weight while I was pregnant that I never put on a stitch of maternity clothes.

Now, someone might wonder what my doctor thought about all of this weight loss during my pregnancy. The only question she ever had was whether I was feeling sick. That was because all of my pregnancy "vital signs" were very healthy during the entire pregnancy. Finally, I went into labor in February of 1998, three weeks early. I was so worried; my first pregnancy went full term and my daughter weighed in at 8 pounds 3 ounces after a C-section. My first thought was that the second baby was coming early because of the weight loss. I could not have been more incorrect. My second child, a boy, weighed in at 6 pounds 9 ounces (three weeks early), was delivered naturally and was healthy. In fact, if my son had gone full term, he probably would have weighed more than 8 pounds. And the most exciting part of all of this was that I actually went into labor weighing four pounds less than when I got pregnant. After all was said and done, I lost 35 pounds while I was pregnant!

Now my son is six months old, I am still nursing him and he is growing like a weed. My weight has remained steady, even though I have started to "cheat" a little. I still want to lose about 20 pounds more, but I decided not to worry about it while I was nursing. That is because for the first time in my 34 years of life, I feel as though I have control over my weight. I cannot put into words what a wonderful feeling it is not to be afraid of food. I do not count calories at all and I never feel hungry. I cannot thank you enough, Suzanne, for sharing this lifestyle with the world. If it were not for Somersizing, there is no doubt that I would still be struggling with my weight. This is the simplest way to melt the pounds away and it truly is a lifesaver.

With much love and affection,
Linda England

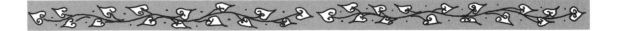

sugar and highly starchy foods to turn to for quick energy sources, our bodies have to look elsewhere to provide us with vital energy . . . and guess where they look first? Our fat reserves!

Our fat reserves become our bodies' vital energy source. That layer of fat starts melting away while we are infused with energy—all the while eating delicious, nutritious foods loaded with flavor.

For those of you who say, "I crave carbohydrates like bread and pasta! And I can't live without a little sugar fix in the afternoon!" I will tell you that these cravings will pass. When I first started Somersizing, my doctor gave me Betafood (a natural herb) to take away sugar cravings. I buy it at the health food store. At first you may feel as though you are making substantial sacrifices by not eating the pasta, pizza, potatoes, cookies, cakes, and candy to which your body may be accustomed. As your system unloads the built-up sugar from your cells, your cravings for these types of sugar and carbohydrates will diminish. Some people *ease* their way into the program by weaning themselves off these foods gradually over the first week or two, until they cut them out completely and then diligently begin Level One on the third week or so. This way they are not asking their bodies to go "cold turkey" away from the sweets and bad carbohydrates that keep them overweight and unhealthy. Others decide to just go for it and begin this new lifestyle full force from day one. I recommend you try the latter.

Either way, I will tell you there is no way to lose weight magically. Nothing is totally free. But the benefits of the Somersize sys-

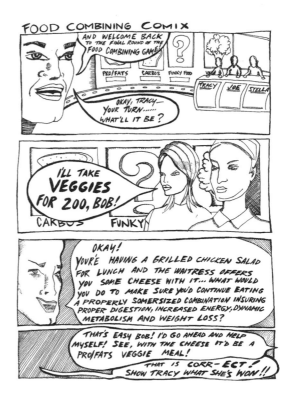

tem far outweigh the restrictions. So I can't eat sugar and white bread . . . look at what I can eat! Whole grains, fresh vegetables, fruit, a huge variety of meats, cheese, and delicious sauces! That's right . . . when I want butter or cream or eggs or cheese, I eat it. Hardly a sacrifice at all to lose all the weight you want, gain vital energy, and keep yourself at your metabolic prime in order to stave off disease.

Soon you will be down to your goal weight and you can begin Level Two, where you incorporate some sugar and starches in moderation without gaining back the weight. Because, come on, every now and then little Suzie Mahoney just has to have a potato . . . so I have it. And I make sure it's really worth it.

SEVEN

The Somersize Program

Now that we've covered the physiology of the program and you understand how crucial it is to eat well, let's get down to the nuts and bolts of what you eat on a day-to-day basis. If you read my first book, *Eat Great, Lose Weight,* you are already familiar with this information; but I urge you to read this section anyway because there are a few pieces of updated material in addition to the simple guidelines of Somersizing.

ELIMINATE

As we've discussed, the most important foods to eliminate are those that cause our blood sugar to fluctuate too much. In addition to sugar and white flour, I have made a list of Funky Foods that cause similar problems.

The first group of Funky Foods is made up of sugar sources. Some are natural and some are refined, but natural or not, they're still sugar, and I avoid them completely when I'm trying to lose weight.

SUGARS

White sugar	Molasses
Brown sugar	Honey
Raw sugar	Maple syrup
Corn syrup	Beets
Sucrose	Carrots
Fructose	

I know it seems weird to eliminate carrots, which have many nutritional qualities, including essential beta-carotene and vitamin A, but carrots are very high in sugar and we get plenty of beta-carotene from broccoli and kale, while vitamin A is found in cantaloupe, peaches, and apricots.

The next group of Funky Foods is made up of foods that are high in starch. These turn directly to sugar (glucose) upon digestion. And remember, we don't need to give

SUGAR ALTERNATIVES: STEVIA—NATURE'S SOLUTION TO SUGAR

Since my last book, I have found a sugar alternative called stevia. Stevia is an herb—Stevia rebaudiana—also known as "honeyleaf." These sweet leaves contain a compound three hundred to four hundred times as sweet as sugar. In South America this herb has been used since the 1500s as a natural sweetener. Today stevia is used as a sweetener and food additive in several countries, including Japan, Paraguay, Brazil, Korea, Thailand, and China. In these countries you may find stevia instead of sugar, saccharin, or aspartame, in products such as candy, ice cream, cookies, sodas, pickles, and chewing gum. Unlike saccharin or aspartame, stevia is all natural, and no negative clinical reports have appeared in any of these countries where stevia is available.

In the United States you can find stevia in health food stores in liquid or powder form. It is a completely sugar-free, zero-calorie, all-natural sweetener that causes no insulin response; an excellent alternative for diabetics, those prone to yeast infections, and, of course, Somersizers. Stevia is extremely concentrated and should be used sparingly to achieve the best taste. Start with just one drop. Some people detect a licoricelike flavor, depending on the potency.

This herb is stable in both hot and acidic conditions, so it can even be used in cooking. Replacing sugar with stevia for baking, however, can be a little tricky. Sugar is the element responsible for browning baked goods, as well as adding volume. When you use stevia instead of sugar, you will need to drastically alter the amount of liquid and dry ingredients. At this point, I have not had much success in creating desserts sweetened with stevia. I will continue testing, but in the meantime, I use a small amount of either sugar or saccharin (for the times on Level One when you just have to have something sweet). Unfortunately I've read far too many controversial medical reports on the dangers of aspartame. In fact, more than 80 percent of all food additive complaints to the FDA are related to aspartame. And frightening studies show that aspartame causes irreversible brain damage in laboratory animals. Even more terrifying, the young and the old are most vulnerable. As I mentioned earlier, one can of diet soda may be enough to raise toxins in the brain of an infant higher than levels that damaged brains of immature animals!

We should put a skull and crossbones on products containing aspartame. Please, find a way to eliminate these chemicals from your life; try Mother Nature's solution—stevia. It's a safe and healthy alternative for those of us with a sweet tooth who don't want the insulin response from sugar or the chemicals from aspartame.

our bodies extra sugar because we can use our fat reserves.

STARCHES

White flour   Yams
White rice   Pumpkin
Corn   Butternut squash
Potatoes   Acorn squash
Sweet potatoes Hubbard squash
Parsnips   Bananas

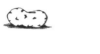

There are so many wonderful alternatives to white flour: whole wheat, pumpernickel, rye, amaranth, spelt, and kamut, to name a few. White rice can be replaced with brown rice, which has a wonderful earthy flavor, or (better yet) wild rice, which has even less starch. As for corn and potatoes, you will be eating greater amounts of green vegetables rather than filling up on starchy vegetables that cause a sugar surge and extra pounds. Think about the fact that corn and potatoes are most often used to fatten up our livestock, and then maybe it won't be so hard to resist that plate of fries! And I know you will be shocked when I tell you to eliminate bananas—how about all that potassium? Sorry, but bananas are very high in sugar, and with all the other fruits you can eat, you won't miss them.

The third group of Funky Foods doesn't seem to fit into any of our four Somersized Food Groups because they contain protein or fat *and* carbohydrates. Take nuts: they are a

Update from
*EAT GREAT,
LOSE WEIGHT*

Parsnips are new to the Funky Foods list. I previously had them grouped with the Veggies, but they are higher in starch than I realized, so they are now officially a Funky Food. They are, however, still a better option than potatoes, so you will see a few recipes including parsnips in Level Two.

protein, they do have fat, *and* they are rich in carbohydrates. Although many of these foods are natural sources of good fats (necessary for cell reproduction), the combination with carbohydrates makes them a no-no for Somersizing purposes in Level One.

BAD COMBO FOODS

Nuts   Coconuts
Olives   Low-fat or whole
Liver   milk and yogurt
Avocados   Tofu

If you are a strict vegetarian and you need additional protein sources, I do make an exception regarding tofu. Although tofu has protein, fat, *and* carbohydrates, I recommend you treat it as a Pro/Fat and combine it only with Veggies.

The last group of Funky Foods is made up of caffeine and alcohol. Just like other funky foods, caffeine can cause highs and lows in your blood sugar, which leads to insulin resistance. I'd hate to see you eat a perfectly combined meal and then blow it with one cup of coffee. Feel free to drink decaffeinated coffee (try Starbucks' delicious Guatemalan decaf) and herbal teas. And don't worry, when you combine correctly you'll have a steady source of energy to get you through the day, rather than experiencing the highs and lows that keep you reaching for caffeine or sweets. As for alcohol, everyone knows it makes you fat, especially beer and hard liquor. Now that you understand the connection between insulin and weight gain around the midsection, a "beer belly" makes perfect sense. Red wine has recently been found to have beneficial effects, and we will incorporate it later on when we are maintaining our weight, but during Level One we will steer clear of all alcohol. I do, however, make an exception with regard to cooking. If you are doing well on Level One, you may use wine in some of my recipes because the alcohol burns off and it leaves a delicious flavor in your cooking.

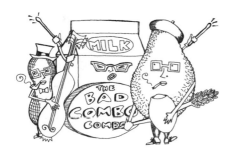

CAFFEINE AND ALCOHOL

Coffee	Beer
Caffeinated teas	Hard alcohol
Caffeinated sodas	Wine
Cocoa	

I know it seems like a strange list of foods to eliminate, but soon it will become second nature. Sugar, starches, bad combo foods, caffeine, and alcohol are all avoided *completely* on Level One. But don't worry, you don't have to say good-bye to these foods forever. They'll be back, in moderation, when we reach our goal weight and advance to Level Two, the maintenance portion of Somersizing.

SEPARATE

In order to learn how to combine our foods in a way that maximizes our digestion, we must first separate foods into our four Somersized Food Groups: Pro/Fats, Carbos, Veggies, and Fruit. Although many foods are made up of a combination of protein, fat, and carbohydrate, we have grouped them by their predominant feature to simplify the program. For instance, *all* the foods found in the Carbos, Veggies, and Fruit groups contain carbohydrates, but the carbohydrate levels vary greatly, which is why I have broken them down into different groups. I have briefly described each group here and have included complete lists of these foods in the Reference Guide (pages 254–256).

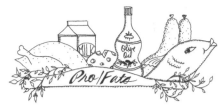

Pro/Fats

The first Somersize group is made up of foods high in protein and/or fat. I put these two food groups together because many of the foods that contain protein also contain fat.

Proteins are made up of organic compounds called amino acids. These amino acids are the building blocks for the human body. Dr. Schwarzbein has helped me see that proteins play a role in virtually every cellular function: they regulate muscle contraction, antibody production, and blood vessel expansion and contraction to maintain normal blood pressure. Protein is a critically important part of the diet because it supplies us with new amino acids that are needed to make these different proteins.

By now you understand the virtues of fat and know that eliminating fat completely from your diet is unhealthy. Fats provide a major storage form of metabolic fuel. When they break down they provide us with energy. Fats also help to facilitate the use of essential fat-soluble vitamins like A, D, E, and K. Vitamin A is necessary for healthy eyes and skin; vitamin D helps to absorb calcium; vitamin E prevents cholesterol deposits; and vitamin K contributes to healthy blood clotting. Fat also helps to stabilize blood sugar. And fat is the body's fuel source that causes the least amount of insulin response. Essential fatty acids cannot

be manufactured by our bodies on their own; they, too, must be included in our daily meals. Unsaturated fats, like olive oil, canola oil, and fish oils, help to lower cholesterol levels and should be included in our meals.

Any of the foods in the Pro/Fats group can be eaten together or in combination with Veggies.

Carbos

Carbohydrates are derived mostly from plant sources rather than from animal sources. Carbos are the primary metabolic fuel in our Westernized diets. As I explained earlier, carbos break down into glucose, which is one of the body's main sources of energy. (The other is fat.) Since we have other mechanisms in our bodies to produce glucose, carbos are the one nutrient not absolutely essential in our diet.

Completely eliminating carbohydrates from our diet is dangerous. On the Somersize system we eliminate *refined* carbohydrates like sugar, white flour, and white rice, but we do enjoy complex carbohydrates like whole-grain pastas and cereals, which still have many essential vitamins and nutrients intact. In addition, complex carbohydrates provide fiber and roughage necessary for the digestive process.

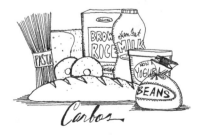

On an emotional level, carbohydrates cause a release of serotonin—the "feel good" hormone. If you are prone to depression, completely eliminating carbohydrates causes a halt in serotonin levels, which can lead to depression. Be careful, however, of loading up on the wrong kinds of carbohydrates if you are depressed and looking for a serotonin fix. "Comfort foods" like macaroni and cheese or a turkey pot pie may give you the serotonin release, but they also bring the ill effects of poorly combined, high-starch meals. Stick to reasonable amounts of the foods listed in the Carbos group and you shouldn't have a problem.

Any of the foods in the Carbos group can be eaten together or in combination with Veggies.

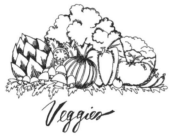

Veggies

All vegetables are technically carbohydrates, but those found in this Somersize category have been chosen because they are low in starch and cause only a minute rise in the blood sugar. Vegetables are packed with vitamins and minerals and provide essential roughage for proper elimination. I implore you, fill up on vegetables! They are an essential part of your daily diet.

Any of the foods in the Veggies group can be eaten together. And since Veggies can easily be digested with either Pro/Fats or Carbos, you may eat them with either group.

Fruit

Fruits are also technically carbohydrates, but because of their unique sugar content, fruits must always be eaten alone. Fruits are a great source of fiber and help to keep the digestive tract moving. They are loaded with nutrients and vitamins, but if you mix fruit with other foods, it can lose its nutritional benefits and upset the digestive process. Fruit turns to acid when combined with other food groups and spoils in the stomach, causing gas and that horrible bloated feeling. Fruit as a supposedly "healthy" option for dessert can ruin a perfectly combined meal. Not only will it make you feel uncomfortable, but it can trap the energy of other foods and cause unnecessary storage of fat. So eat fruit . . . please eat fruit. But eat it alone to get the maximum benefits.

As far as fruit juice is concerned, most of the vital nutrients have been pressed out of the fruit by the time it is turned into juice. The remaining juice is mostly fruit sugar. Therefore I recommend you eat the whole fruit to receive the fiber and drink fruit

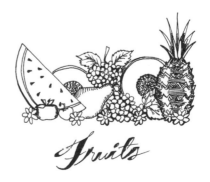

juice sparingly. Concentrated fruit juice is often used as a sugar substitute. Unfortunately your body reacts exactly the same to fruit sugar as it does to regular sugar; it makes insulin spike. During Level One beware of overindulging on all-fruit-juice-sweetened sorbet or frozen fruit bars, even though they are technically *all* fruit. Remember, in Level One we are trying to heal our insulin resistance and these types of treats can set us back. The same goes for dried fruit; the sugar concentration becomes far more intense with dried fruits. I suggest they be eaten rarely, if at all, on Level One.

Here are some guidelines on how you can eat delicious and nutritious fresh fruit and gain all the benefits without creating digestion problems:

Eat Fruit on an empty stomach.

Eat Fruit alone, then wait twenty minutes and you may follow up with a Carbo meal. (The twenty-minute lead time gets the digestion of the fruit going and eliminates problem combinations.)

Eat Fruit alone, then wait one hour and you may follow up with a Pro/Fats meal.

If you want Fruit for a snack or for dessert, you must wait two hours after your last meal to avoid any problems.

Dried fruit, fruit juice, and fruit juice concentrate should be used sparingly on Level One.

Any of the foods in the Fruit group can be eaten together.

Free Foods

There are a few items that may be combined with Pro/Fats, Veggies, or Carbos because they do not conflict with any of the food groups. These include soy sauce, vinegar, mustard, herbs, and spices. In addition, lemons and limes, though technically fruits, are very low in sugar and therefore may be used to flavor any of the four Somersized Food Groups.

THE GLYCEMIC INDEX

All carbohydrates will break down into sugar upon digestion. But as we've dis-

A SOMERSIZING SUCCESS STORY

Dear Suzanne,

Thank you for your wonderful "Somersize" eating plan. Although in my younger years I never had a weight problem, I found, like you, that as I was approaching my fifties my metabolism had slowed down dramatically. No matter how much I exercised or how many dollars I spent on so-called Miracle Herbal Fat Burns, the only fat I lost was in my wallet.

I also have Crohn's disease; and after five surgeries, I still have only half of a normal digestive tract. So, obviously, I also have to be careful about what I eat.

One day about eight weeks ago, I was complaining to a co-worker that I had been suffering for several days from indigestion and was afraid that perhaps an old ulcer had once again surfaced. She told me about the Somersize program and loaned me her book. After reading your book, it made so much sense that I decided to buy my own copy and immediately began your program. If nothing else, I thought it would help my digestion.

The only hardship for me was to give up my nightly martini after work. But I was determined to shed these ten extra pounds. Well, it was incredible. I started to feel more energetic after just two days and lost 4 pounds in five days. After 10 days, I was down 7 pounds, and then dropped down 9 pounds in just three weeks. I am now down 13 pounds and can't believe how wonderful I feel. I work out only twice a week because of my schedule (I'm a finance director for a large GM dealership in San Jose, California). And yet I have lost 3 inches in my waist.

Now, when people ask what I'm doing, I have become one of your biggest advocates and show them your book. My fiancé is so proud of the way I look; but the best part is that I look in the mirror and am proud, too.

Well, I just wanted to share my wonderful results with you and thank you again for making me feel young again.

Sincerely,
Alba Manasseri

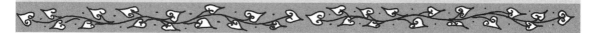

cussed, some carbohydrates create a much larger insulin response than others. Although I do not ask you to calculate calories, fat grams, sugars, or even carbohydrates as part of the Somersize program, I am including the Glycemic Index Chart on page 48 to assist you in seeing the effects of various kinds of carbohydrates. The glycemic index rises corresponding to the level of hyperglycemia caused by eating carbohydrates. The higher the glycemic index, the higher the level of hyperglycemia.

You will notice that foods in their natural state have a lower glycemic index than foods that have been processed. Whole-wheat

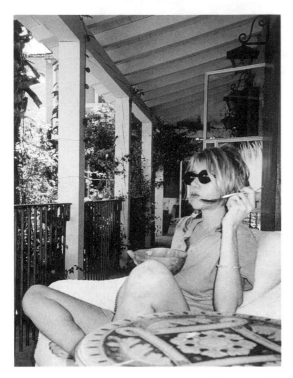

Enjoying my first course for breakfast on the porch (one half of a perfect, delicious cantaloupe).

bread breaks down into less glucose than its processed counterpart, white bread. Brown rice has a lower glycemic index than its refined counterpart, white rice. This is owing largely to the fiber content of foods. The greater the fiber, the lower the glycemic index.

Fruits and vegetables are also carbohydrates, with varying degrees of glucose potential. Seeing how they rate on the glycemic index will help to explain how I divided all food into my four Somersized Food Groups. Those vegetables with the highest glycemic index, such as potatoes,

beets, and carrots, have been labeled Funky Foods and eliminated altogether. Whole grains, beans, and dairy products have a moderate glycemic index and have been categorized in the Somersize Carbo Food Group. And nonstarchy vegetables with the lowest glycemic index have been categorized in the Somersize Veggies Food Group.

GLYCEMIC INDEX CHART

Beer	110
Glucose	100
White bread	95
Instant potatoes	95
Honey	90
Jam	90
Cornflakes	85
Popcorn	85
Carrots	85
Potatoes	70
Pasta (from white flour)	65
Bananas	60
Dried fruit	60
Brown rice	50
Whole-wheat bread	50
Whole-wheat pasta	45
Fresh white beans	40
Oatmeal	40
Whole-rye bread	40
Green peas	40
Whole cereals	35
Dairy products	35
Wild rice	35
Fresh fruit	35
Dried beans	30
Dark chocolate	22
Soy	15
Green vegetables	Less than 15

WHAT'S THE DEAL WITH DAIRY?

Many people, including me, get confused about dairy products with regards to Somersizing. When you're having a Pro/Fats meal, you may eat all the cheese you want and you may add cream to your sauce, but you can't use a splash of milk in your decaf coffee. When you're having a Carbos meal you can eat nonfat yogurt, but you can't use nonfat yogurt with a Pro/Fats meal. What's the deal? Let me help to clarify this issue.

Milk has protein and carbohydrates, whether it's nonfat, low-fat, or whole milk. Yogurt has protein and carbohydrates, whether it's nonfat, low-fat, or whole-milk yogurt. When we eat proteins or fats, we do not eat foods that contain carbohydrates; therefore, we cannot include any kind of milk or yogurt in the Pro/Fats meal. When we eat a Carbos meal, we can include products with protein, as long as they do not contain any fat. Therefore, we can include nonfat milk and nonfat yogurt. Low-fat and whole milk or yogurt are grouped as Funky Foods because they have fat and carbohydrates.

What about cream, butter, cheese, sour cream, and the like? These "milk" products have a very different quality than their plain milk or yogurt cousins. In the process of making cream, butter, or cheese, all the carbohydrates are processed out of these dairy products, leaving only the protein and fat. That is the reason why these dairy products without *carbohydrates are included in the Pro/Fats group, while the milk products* with *carbohydrates are grouped in the Carbos group.*

Get it? If not, read it again.

DAIRY PRODUCTS

PRO/FATS—DAIRY PRODUCTS WITHOUT CARBOHYDRATES	CARBOS—DAIRY PRODUCTS WITH CARBOHYDRATES AND NO FAT	FUNKY FOODS— DAIRY PRODUCTS WITH CARBOHYDRATES AND FAT
Butter	Nonfat milk	Low-fat milk
Cream	Nonfat yogurt	Whole milk
Cheese	Nonfat cheese	Low-fat yogurt
Sour cream		Whole-milk yogurt
Crème fraîche		

EIGHT

Let's Get Started—Level One

Now that you have a basic understanding of what foods to eliminate and how to categorize the rest into our four Somersized Food Groups, you can get started on your new lifestyle. Let me walk you through each meal so you can see how easy it is to Somersize at every meal.

BREAKFAST

Each meal is an opportunity to eat something great, even on Level One when you're trying to lose weight. Let's talk about all the delicious breakfast options. I love breakfast! Cereal, toast, fruit, eggs, bacon, sausage . . . bring them on! As long as you follow the Somersize combinations, you may eat *any* of those foods for breakfast, just not in the same sitting. Here are your choices:

Breakfast #1—Fruit meal
Breakfast #2—Carbos meal
Breakfast #3—Fruit, wait twenty
   minutes, then Carbos meal
Breakfast #4—Pro/Fats and Veggies
   meal

Breakfast #1—Fruit Meal

Start your day off with a couple of plums, an orange, or half a cantaloupe. Or combine your favorite fruits in a blender with some juice and a few ice cubes for a frosty fruit smoothie. Or dice some mangoes, pineapple, papaya, and grapes for a tasty fruit salad. Remember, you may eat any kind of fruit, except bananas, which are a Funky Food. Fruit is best in the morning when eaten on an empty stomach. Fruit keeps you regular and is loaded with vitamins, nutrients, and a natural source of energy.

Breakfast #2 — Carbos Meal

Morning is the best time of the day to eat your Carbos because you can use the natural energy they supply throughout the day. There are a number of wonderful options to satisfy your hunger. I like whole-grain toast with nonfat cottage cheese or yogurt. Or I like hot or cold whole-grain cereal with nonfat milk. Since we cannot combine any fat with our Carbos, this is the only time we choose fat-free products, specifically nonfat dairy products. I guard against choosing *processed* fat-free dairy products, like fat-free cream cheese, because they are often loaded with starches, fillers, and chemicals.

Remember, you may have Veggies with your Carbos, so feel free to top your toast with tomato and basil or a slice of red onion, if you like.

Breakfast #3 — Fruit, Wait Twenty Minutes, Then Carbos Meal

Fruit, then Carbos, is my favorite choice for breakfast because these foods provide me with necessary fiber and a host of vitamins and nutrients. Besides that, they just taste good! Alan is the master breakfast maker in our home. Usually he brings me a great fruit smoothie in the morning. Then I work out with my son-in-law, Frank, who is my personal trainer. Afterward we have cereal with nonfat milk, toast, and decaf coffee. Morning is the best time to eat your Fruit and Carbos so that you have plenty of time to burn off the natural sources of energy they provide.

Breakfast #4 — Pro/Fats and Veggies Meal

In a Pro/Fats and Veggies breakfast you may have anything from the Pro/Fats group with anything from the Veggies group. You have so many choices with this breakfast. The "incredible egg" can be scrambled, fried, boiled, poached, or made into an omelet or a frittata. Cook the eggs in butter or oil and serve them with sausage or bacon (I look for brands with no nitrates). Or try Alan's Fried Eggs in Onion Nests (page 115). For additional flavor you can even cook your eggs in the bacon or sausage grease. Some diet, huh? You can have meat, fish, or poultry, including chicken, shrimp, crab, lox, and smoked fish. Feel free to add some cheese to that omelet! And don't forget your Veggies, like onions, tomatoes, zucchini, spinach, mushrooms, asparagus, and more.

Any of these foods would make up a perfectly combined Somersized breakfast, so you may eat until you are full. This is a great breakfast option when you're eating out because there are so few restrictions. Just stay away from toast, jelly, potatoes, and fruit with your Pro/Fats and Veggies breakfast.

(If you want to start this meal with Fruit, you must wait one hour until you have your Pro/Fats and Veggies.)

LUNCH AND DINNER

For lunch today, and every day, we are serving salads, soups, sandwiches, chicken, steak, fish, pasta, and more! You just have to decide what food group you feel like and then design a meal in the proper Somersize combination. Here are your choices:

Lunch or Dinner #1—Pro/Fats and Veggies meal
Lunch or Dinner #2—Carbos and Veggies meal
Lunch or Dinner #3—Single Food Group meal

Lunch or Dinner #1— Pro/Fats and Veggies Meal

Flavor, flavor, flavor! That's what you can look forward to with every Pro/Fats and Veggies meal. Meat, poultry, or fish can be grilled, broiled, baked, roasted, or fried and served with plenty of fresh vegetables, raw, steamed, sautéed, or grilled. Enjoy cooking with oil or butter, and don't forget to add the cheese! Preparing meals for yourself at home or eating in a restaurant is a pleasure with the Pro/Fats and Veggies meal. Just watch out for hidden sugars or starches often used in sauces.

Your Pro/Fats and Veggies meals will range from the incredibly simple to the luxuriously extravagant. With so much to choose from, you won't ever get bored eating the same old thing. In fact, your food will probably taste better than ever as you trim your way down to your ideal body weight.

Lunch or Dinner #2— Carbos and Veggies Meal

I choose this option very infrequently, because I prefer to eat my Carbos only in the morning when I'm trying to lose weight. But every now and then you just need a carbohydrate fix at lunch or dinner, and it really hits the spot. You can have any whole grains or beans with nonfat dairy products and any of the vegetables in the Veggies list. Be careful when you look for whole-wheat products . . . many manufacturers are now listing "wheat flour" for regular white flour. It must say "*whole*-wheat flour" to really be a whole grain. In general, if it looks too white to be whole wheat . . . it probably is.

Try brown rice with peas or black bean chili with fresh tomato salsa and whole-wheat tortillas or whole-grain pasta with tomato basil sauce or whole-wheat pita bread with hummus, baba ganoush, and fresh vegetables. With any of these meals you could have a green salad. The key to the Carbos and Veggies meal is to make sure there is absolutely no fat.

This is a very satisfying and healthy option with all the whole grains and fresh vegetables. It can be a little restrictive, however, because on Level One you can't have any fat and you must watch for hidden sugars and Funky Foods. Because this meal is more difficult when you're eating in a restaurant, I normally prepare Carbos and Veggies at home.

Lunch or Dinner #3— Single Food Group Meal

Every now and then you might want to have a meal made up of only one food group, like the all Fruit meal or the all Veggies meal. Of course, this is perfectly fine on

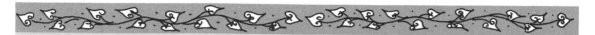

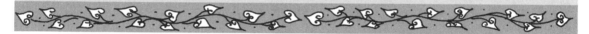

rare occasions, but I do not recommend it with any frequency.

Until you become familiar with your options for breakfast, lunch, and dinner, refer back to this section, or use the convenient Reference Guide on pages 254–256.

FINDING A RHYTHM THAT WORKS

When I'm losing weight on Level One, I find that the fewer carbohydrates I eat, the more results I see. As I explained earlier, carbohydrates are an energy source, and if you're not giving your body many sources of energy, it will have to break down your fat reserves and use *them* as energy. But we don't want to cut out carbohydrates completely because they are an important source of fiber and help keep your system moving properly. And if you go too low with carbohydrates, your body will break down its protein, instead of its fat reserves, to be used as energy.

Here's what works best for me. I like to have the Fruit, then Carbos breakfast. Because carbohydrates are a good energy source, it's best to eat them in the morning so that you can use that energy throughout the day. For lunch or dinner I find more options with Pro/Fats and plenty of Veggies. Carbo meals for lunch and dinner are a little more restrictive because you can have absolutely no fat.

My recommendation is that for breakfast you usually have Breakfast #3—Fruit, then Carbos. For lunch and dinner I recommend Pro/Fats and Veggies as a rule, with the Carbo and Veggies meal as the exception. If you eat too many carbohydrates, even the right kinds of carbohydrates, they could get stored as fat for later use. (And if you're filling up on carbohydrates, you're probably not supplying your body with enough protein and fat.) Remember, your body gets the small amount of carbohydrates it needs because your Pro/Fats and Veggies meals include some carbohydrates in the form of the many vegetables you'll be enjoying. In fact, you could choose the Pro/Fats and Veggies meal at *every* meal and enjoy great

health—it's a perfect combination of protein, fat, and carbohydrates (in the form of low-starch vegetables). This combination gives your body all the essential building materials it needs to thrive. The Carbos and Veggies meal gives you some diversity now and then and, as I said, includes all that great fiber.

This is only a blueprint of how I divide my Pro/Fat and Carbo meals. I find that those carbohydrates tend to fatten me up like a corn-fed cow. However, you may discover that your body can handle more carbohydrates and that you feel better eating mostly grains and vegetables. On the other hand, if you are eating mostly Pro/Fats, you must balance your meals with plenty of fresh vegetables. It is unwise to eat only meat and cheese without the fiber and nutrients added from vegetables.

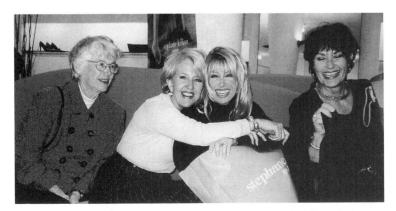

Another of our famous lunches with the Birthday Club, Auntie Helen, my sister Maureen, my sister-in-law Mardi.

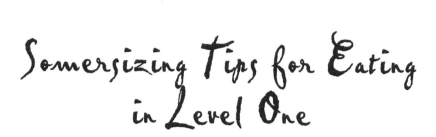

Somersizing Tips for Eating in Level One

I realize this information may seem a bit overwhelming at first, but soon you will discover how simple Somersizing can be. Whenever my friends and family first start the program, they frequently call me with questions. And since I can't give my home phone number to everyone, I have compiled some helpful tips for dining out and eating at home.

TIPS FOR DINING OUT

So many people tell me, "I eat two to three of my meals each day in restaurants; it's impossible to lose weight." Once you understand Somersizing, eating in any restaurant is truly easy. First I scan the menu and decide if I want to choose a Pro/Fats and Veggies meal or a Carbos and Veggies meal. Ninety-five percent of the time I'll choose a Pro/Fats meal, which might be a

green salad with dressing of my choice, a chicken, meat, or fish entrée with a lovely sauce and plenty of steamed, sautéed, or grilled vegetables. On the rare occasion that I choose to have a Carbos and Veggies meal, I might order a vegetarian sandwich on whole-grain bread or brown rice with steamed vegetables and soy sauce.

The key to the Pro/Fats meal is no bread, pasta, potatoes, or rice. We are accustomed to beginning every meal in a restaurant by emptying a basket of bread into our bellies before we even order! Then we eat a meal of meat with potatoes, or a turkey sandwich, or a Chinese chicken salad piled high with fried rice noodles and wontons. Add a couple of glasses of caffeine, like iced tea or diet cola, and you have a recipe for metabolic disaster. These are the things that throw your system into chaos.

You'll be surprised at how quickly you'll get over missing the starch. Make sure to watch for hidden sugars or starches in the salad dressings or sauces. Drill your server a little to get the information you need; make sure your entrée is not dusted with flour before being pan-fried and ask the kitchen to substitute the starchy side dish for extra vegetables or salad. Just make sure all the vegetables are on the Veggies list. It does you no good to get a big side dish of sautéed carrots. And it's a terrible waste of food to be served items you know you cannot eat. (I have a friend who always tells the server she's diabetic to make sure they *really* check for sugar.)

You will also have to get over that feeling of being "overstuffed" when you finish a meal. I used to think I was not full until my stomach became distended and I could not consider putting another bite into my mouth. When you Somersize you will not get that overstuffed feeling because your body is not fighting with bad food combinations that cause digestive problems. Your system becomes cleansed, and you become accustomed to feeling satisfied without feeling stuffed.

The Level One Carbos meal is much more restrictive when you're eating out. It must be fat-free so that all those carbohydrates are burned off rather than stored as fat. Also, watch out for sugars and hidden Funky Foods, and avoid anything from the Pro/Fats group; meat and cheese on that sandwich would throw your system into a tizzy. Even mayonnaise, oil, and avocado are not okay on Level One.

With minimal effort you can enjoy dining at any restaurant and still lose weight. And it's worth it! Judge for yourself. I guar-antee you'll like the way you feel when you Somersize. Neither bloating nor gas, with improved elimination and more energy than ever before.

TIPS FOR EATING AT HOME

As far as eating at home, if you're used to prepared foods, you will need to make some adjustments. Most prepared foods are made with processed products like sugar, white flour, and a variety of unpronounce-able chemicals. Say good-bye to Hamburger Helper! With a little preparation you can learn to create fresh foods that taste much better and are far more nutritious. I keep my refrigerator stocked with ingredients that allow me to prepare meals quickly. I like to shop at our local farmer's market on Saturdays and stock up for the week. Alan and I make a morning of it. We each grab a couple of straw bags and scan the market for the selections of the season. Alan heads straight for the fruit growers—succulent melons, crisp apples, peaches, berries, pomegranates, whatever the season brings. I gravitate toward the vegetable stands. My friend at the mushroom stand will put together a brown bag with his prized shiitake and oyster mushrooms. The lettuce growers display a variety of romaine, endive, radicchio, frisee, baby spinach, but-ter lettuce, and more. I pick up a bag of sugar snap peas, broccoli, cauliflower, green beans, asparagus, onions, leeks, and vine-ripened tomatoes—all grown organically without pesticides.

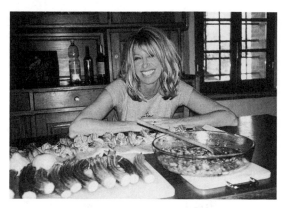

My beautiful stuffed zucchini flowers in a Tuscan kitchen.

On Sundays I do a little cooking; perhaps I'll make some mushroom sausage stuffing with my shiitakes and stuff a small turkey. The next day I'll use the leftover meat for turkey salad served in lettuce cups, and then I'll take the carcass and make a delicious turkey-and-vegetable soup for the following night.

Having ingredients in the house makes coming home from work and preparing dinner so easy. Most of the recipes in this book are quick and require minimal skills as a chef. The most important part of any good recipe is finding good, quality ingredients. You'll find when you shop that you'll mostly buy foods from the perimeter of the grocery store. Start in the produce section for all your fresh fruits and vegetables. Then head for the meat and fish section. Try to look for a great butcher who sells meat without added hormones, nitrates, or preservatives. Go to the bakery to look for fresh bread or bagels made from whole grains. Then stock up in the dairy department on butter, sour

cream, cheese, nonfat milk, and yogurt. I always feel good at the checkout stand when I unload my groceries because I'll have several wrapped packages from the butcher, a ton of baggies from the produce section, and a great selection of cheeses and dairy products. There are no boxes of cookies, crackers, or snack food. It's all *real* food, as close to its natural state as possible.

To give you an idea of what I shop for each week, I've listed some of the ingredients I always like to have in my refrigerator and pantry.

Whole-Grain Bread—whole wheat, pumpernickel, rye; whatever kind you like. Keep an extra loaf in the freezer so you never run out. Check for hidden sugars, fats, fruits, or sweeteners. Choose totally natural breads made without honey or white flour or fruit juice. Again, make sure you look for *whole* wheat, not just *wheat* flour. Many manufacturers are listing white flour now as wheat flour to make you think it is a healthier product. Don't be fooled. White flour begins with a grain of wheat . . . it just gets processed so extensively that none of the nutrients of the original wheat remain in the end product. Sometimes it's difficult to find bread that fits all these requirements. Ask your local bakery if they make all whole-wheat bread. Flat breads are excellent choices and readily available: whole-wheat pita, whole-wheat lavash bread, and whole-wheat tortillas. Just make sure they're made without any fats.

Whole-Grain Pastas—Some whole-wheat pastas can be mushy, so you may have to try a few out. I like De Cecco brand whole wheat best. Whatever brand you choose, look for whole-wheat or durum whole-wheat semolina. I also like whole-wheat and artichoke pasta. Straight semolina on its own is not allowed. Also try pastas made from whole grains like kamut, spelt, or brown rice. Don't forget whole-wheat wonton wrappers for homemade ravioli.

Hot Cereals—Try oatmeal and Cream of Wheat.

Cold Cereals—I like Shredded Wheat, Grape-Nuts, and Crispy Brown Rice. Again, check carefully for sugars and Funky Foods on the labels.

Nonfat Cottage Cheese—Great on your toast in the morning or for a snack in the afternoon.

Nonfat Yogurt—A good-quality plain nonfat yogurt is a delicious treat. Pavel's is my favorite brand, but it's sometimes hard to find.

Nonfat Milk—I buy the kind from farms that don't use any hormones, pesticides, or antibodies.

Beans—Use dried, canned, or fresh. I like cannellini beans, pinto beans, lentils, black-eyed peas, and garbanzo beans (also called chickpeas).

Mustard—Pick up a variety of yellow, whole grain, and Dijon.

Rice—Choose brown rice and wild rice. Make sure neither is blended with white rice of any sort.

Phyllo Dough—Many types are whole wheat. Keep a box in the freezer for quick Level Two tarts and pastries.

Cheese—Buy whatever kind you like. I always have buffalo mozzarella and goat cheese in the fridge. I also try to keep Stilton or another good blue, Romano, and feta on hand. My favorite Parmesan is Parmigiano-Reggiano. Pecorino is wonderful, and sometimes I splurge on a triple cream like Camembert or Brie. On most diets celery is the only "free" food that can be eaten at will. Who knew cheese could keep you so lean and healthy! Keep little individually wrapped cheeses, like string cheese or Laughing Cow, on hand for snacks.

Butter—There's nothing like the real flavor of butter. I keep salted and sweet on hand.

Fresh Eggs—I get mine from the farmer's market for the freshest of fresh. I like to keep some hard boiled in the fridge for quick snacks.

Mayonnaise—Best Foods or Hellmann's is my favorite brand. I used to avoid it in Level One because it has sugar listed in the ingredient list. But if you look on the label, you'll notice there are zero carbohydrates per serving. I presume the added sugar must be in trace amounts or there would be an increased carbohydrate listing. So enjoy your Best Foods, or make your own with my easy recipe from *Eat Great, Lose Weight.*

Fresh Seafood—I always buy my seafood the same day I eat it. My favorites are sea bass, trout, tuna, shrimp, and scallops. The exception are frozen Alaskan king crab legs. They're expensive, but an amazing treat and a cinch to make.

Meat—I like to keep a few packages in the freezer to thaw for a quick meal. Pork chops, lean ground beef, steaks, and lamb chops. Remember, the fat in meat is *real* fat, which promotes healthy cells.

Oil—I buy extra-virgin olive oil by the case. I use it in almost every meal. I also keep safflower or canola oil. And don't forget peanut oil, hot chili oil, and sesame oil to flavor those delicious Asian meals.

Vinegar—Balsamic, red wine, white wine, and champagne vinegar are my household staples. Rice vinegar is good to have around for Asian dishes.

Poultry—I eat a lot of chicken. I have the butcher make a few packages with two chicken breasts in each. That way I can keep them in the freezer and thaw them quickly for an easy meal. Same with turkey cutlets—they're a nice alternative with a slightly different flavor. I also keep ground chicken and ground turkey on hand.

Lettuce—I buy my lettuce on the weekend and completely wash, dry, and bag it so that I have easy salads all week long (or I buy prewashed lettuce). I like red leaf, butter lettuce, romaine, radicchio, and endive.

Onions—I love onions: brown, red, scallions, and leeks. You'll see from my recipes, I can make any meal great by starting with onions!

Garlic—and plenty of it. Sometimes I peel a few heads and keep the cloves in olive oil in the fridge for quick access.

Ginger—Fresh and ground for Asian recipes.

Soy Sauce—For Asian recipes.

Fresh Veggies—Buy whatever is in season and looks great: asparagus, broccoli, cauliflower, tomatoes, summer squash, zucchini, fennel, celery, celery root, green beans, bell peppers, and so on. You'll be eating lots of vegetables to make up for the missing starch, so load up.

Canned Goods—I always keep canned tomatoes on hand for easy-to-prepare sauces. I buy tomato sauce, crushed tomatoes, and whole peeled tomatoes. I also like hearts of palm, which are great in salads. Canned bamboo shoots are good for Asian dishes, and a few cans of tuna fish are nice to have around to throw into salads. And I always keep cans of chicken and beef stock on hand for the times when I can't make my own (check for hidden sugars or starches). Hain is my favorite brand because it has no preservatives and it tastes great.

Frozen Veggies—I use frozen veggies only when I absolutely can't get them fresh. The flavor doesn't compare.

Fresh and Dried Herbs—Basil, thyme, rosemary, parsley, tarragon, dill, mint, and cilantro are a few that I always like to have around. Most of these are easy to grow yourself if you have a sunny spot.

Fresh Fruits—I choose whatever is in season: apples, grapes, mangoes, papaya, melons, berries, citrus fruits, and more. Remember, because their sugar content is so low, lemons and limes can be used to season foods from any of the four Somersize Food Groups.

Frozen Fruits—Always great for fruit smoothies and Level Two pastries. I make sure to have frozen berries, peaches, pineapple, papaya, and mango when I can find them.

WHAT TO DRINK?

Water. I highly recommend you drink eight to ten glasses of water a day. But try not to drink *with* your meals because water can dilute your digestive juices, which slows down the digestive process. Your stomach acids are strongest right before you begin a new meal. When you eat, the acids break down the food quickly and pass it from the stomach. If you drink a big glass of water before your meal, these gastric juices become diluted and are less effective at breaking down the food. Therefore if you must drink with your meal, eat a portion of your food before you drink anything so as not to dilute the strength of the gastric juices. It's best to drink your eight to ten glasses between meals. Besides water, you can also have decaffeinated coffee, teas, and even diet sodas, if you must. Personally I stay away from soft drinks, and you already know why: they are loaded with dangerous chemicals. You would be doing your body a favor to eliminate them as well.

DON'T SKIP MEALS

Whether you're eating at home or dining in restaurants, make sure not to skip meals. Our mothers always told us that breakfast is the most important meal of the day, right? In many ways they were correct. Your body has been fasting while you sleep so when you wake up in the morning you have gone for some eight to ten hours without food. If you skip breakfast and don't eat until lunch, your body has gone for twelve to fourteen hours without food. When you finally eat lunch, your body's survival instinct kicks in. It doesn't know when you're going to feed it again, so it hangs on to every morsel instead of processing the food properly. Remember to eat at least three meals a day—or eat several smaller meals throughout the day if you prefer.

PORTION CONTROL

People often ask me about portion size because they are used to feeling deprived on diets. Somersizing does not require you to measure any of your foods. You simply eat until you are full. At first you may need to eat more food to feel satisfied because you are accustomed to having that "stuffed" feeling when you finish a meal. You will not feel "stuffed" or bloated when you eat in proper combinations. I don't worry about you eating *too* much; it is difficult to overeat when you are eating only nutritious foods, because your body will signal you when it is sated. Overeating junk food, however, is a cinch, because you can eat and eat and eat without ever giving your body what it needs to thrive! Your body may keep sending hunger messages until you give it the nutritious food it craves.

GET MOVING!

Exercise is an important part of any weight loss program. That doesn't mean you have to spend three hours a day taking aerobics classes. I realize that not everyone has the time or the money to join a gym and work out every day. I know with my busy schedule that it's hard to find the time to exercise regularly. When I'm home I try to work out as much as I can with my son-in-law, Frank Buffa. Alan's daughter, Leslie, has been married to Frank for four years. He is the former Mr. France and the best personal trainer I've ever worked with. I especially like our workouts when he brings our darling granddaughter, Daisy, along.

Frank comes to our house in the morning and takes Alan and me through a workout of resistance training. I can't tell you what a difference it has made in my muscle tone! Just thirty minutes a day, three times a week (except when I travel). My arms are no longer floppy, my tummy is tightening, and my backside is getting higher and higher.

Somersizing helps me stay at the right weight, while exercising helps me keep the right shape. And it makes you feel great! Just make sure that you're giving your body the protein and fat it needs to build muscle while you're exercising. A low-fat, high-carbohydrate diet in combination with strenuous exercise is a recipe for disaster. Your muscles and bones can deteriorate without the proper nutrients to keep them healthy and strong.

Get yourself out and start moving. My motto is, "Be fit, not fanatic." On the days when you just cannot find time for a workout, take a walk, just a twenty-minute walk,

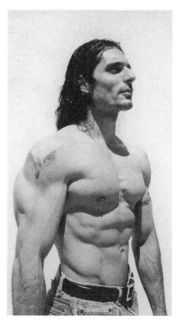

My son-in-law and my trainer, Frank Buffa (who was Mr. France), and he's nice, too!

in the morning or the afternoon. Play tag with your kids. Take the stairs instead of the elevator. Take an active look at your activity level. Exercise helps you build lean muscle mass, which is a key element in losing weight. Lean muscle mass helps you burn calories twenty-four hours a day.

Plus, exercise is another way to keep insulin levels balanced. It helps us release the stored sugar from our cells so that we can get down to burning our fat reserves and losing that extra weight. Find an activity that brings you enjoyment; it doesn't have to cost money—it just has to get you breathing a little harder.

BE DILIGENT!

As long as you are following *all* the Level One guidelines, you may eat until you are full and still lose weight. Be diligent! You cannot Somersize halfheartedly. Your body is in the process of healing as it unloads years of stored-away sugar in its cells. In order to retrain your body to burn your fat reserves, you must not confuse it by slipping up with bad combinations or Funky Foods. Besides, you have so many choices, there is no need to slip up. You will love eating this way and seeing the amazing results. Some people see results immediately and lose five or more pounds in the first week. Others don't see results until the second, third, or even fourth week. Be patient! You body is detoxifying from all the sugar and chemicals and bad combinations to which it has become accustomed. You *will* see results, and once it begins you'll start to melt away down to your ideal body weight. Best of all, you'll love eating this way!

I have synthesized all the information you need to know for Level One in the Reference Guide (pages 254–256) at the back of the book. Use this guide as a reminder of which foods belong in what categories. In no time you will get the hang of Somersizing and it will all become second nature.

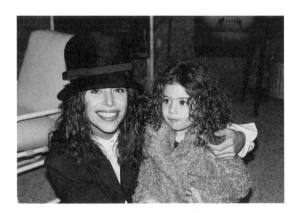

My great stepdaughter Leslie and our granddaughter Daisy.

TEN

Living Lean—Level Two

After you've lost the extra weight and made it down to your goal weight, you're ready for the maintenance portion of Somersizing, which I call Level Two. By this time you are looking and feeling great. You have trained your pancreas not to oversecrete insulin by eliminating Funky Foods. And rather than filling up on empty carbohydrates that give your body a quick source of energy, you have trained your body to use your fat reserves as an energy source. You've conditioned your system to digest quickly and efficiently by cutting out bad combina-

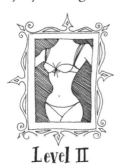

Level II

tions. You have released the stored sugar from your cells and healed your metabolism. Now your body is in great shape and can handle a few imbalances.

The last thing we want is for you to throw away all your hard work by resuming old habits. Level Two is about helping you find a balance so you can enjoy previously forbidden foods in moderation, without completely throwing caution to the wind. Much of the information in the following sections is similar to the first *Eat Great, Lose Weight* book. But please take the time to read them anyway because new information is peppered throughout.

In Level Two *you* are the only person who can determine how much imbalance your body can handle. Some people have to stay very close to Level One guidelines, with a minor imbalance here and there, in order to maintain their weight. Others find they can create quite a few imbalances and still maintain their weight. By a process of trial and error you will soon know how many imbalances your body can handle. I know when I've created too much of an imbalance when I feel bloated after a meal. Another warning for me is if I feel tired an hour or two after a meal. These are signs that I have wandered too far from Level One and need to pull in the reins. Of course, the most obvious sign is if you start to gain weight. Then you know you need to cut back on the treats and get back to eating cheese!

There are specific guidelines necessary to lose weight in Level One, and if you've gotten down to your goal weight, you have followed them diligently. I wish I could give you specific guidelines for Level Two, but actually that's the beauty of it . . . there are no hard-and-fast rules for Level Two. You are in control of your body, and you need to find a rhythm you can live with for the rest of your life.

The great thing is that no matter how large an imbalance you create, you can always find your equilibrium. Level Two is really an extension of Level One, with a few indulgences here and there. Of course, moderation is the key to maintaining your weight. I find that if I eat a Level One lunch, like a Cobb salad with chicken, cheese, bacon, green onions, and tomatoes, every now and then I can add a piece of whole-grain bread without upsetting my system too much. Or if I want to indulge myself a little more, I might hold the bread and maybe have a piece of flourless chocolate cake. Certainly I would not have chocolate cake every day or it would catch up with me. And I would not eat the Cobb salad with the wheat bread *and* the cake because that would be more carbohydrates than I could handle. Of course, a Cobb salad with a *white* flour roll and the cake would make me bloat city.

I also find on Level Two that I can handle a few more Carbos and Veggies meals. Whereas in Level One I almost exclusively eat my Carbos at breakfast, on Level Two I might incorporate a few lunches and dinners revolving around whole-wheat pasta or brown rice. Again, only you can determine how many of these Carbos meals you can eat without upsetting your system.

MIXING PRO/FATS AND CARBOS

As your system becomes clean you will find that your body can handle a small amount of carbohydrate *with* your Pro/Fats meal. When you combine carbohydrate with Pro/Fats, stay within the Carbos list. For instance, you might add one slice of buttered whole-wheat toast with your eggs in the morning, but a stack of pancakes made from white flour would be overdoing it. Or you could have a tuna melt on one slice of whole-grain bread for lunch, but the side of potato salad would not be advised. For dinner you might have a small portion of wild rice with your chicken and vegetables, but a side of white pasta would be a bit much.

Every now and then you may really want those pancakes or potato salad or pasta. Just make sure the imbalance is worth it to you. Then go back and eat a few strict Level One meals for a while until you rebalance your

A SOMERSIZING SUCCESS STORY

Dear Suzanne,

I was very happy and excited to speak to you last month when you were on the Home Shopping Club to share with you my success with the Somersizing Plan.

I was diagnosed with hypothyroidism seven years ago at the age of 39. I had put on 20 pounds and felt sluggish and tired. Since that time, I have tried joining Weight Watchers and after four months of totally sticking with their plan, had lost a total of .6 pound. That's not even one pound.

I then tried Richard Simmons's Deal-A-Meal along with a new exercise program. After four months I had lost three pounds, so of course I became discouraged and gave up.

In May of this year I purchased your plan on the Home Shopping Network and by my target date of July 26th (I was going on vacation and had to wear a swimsuit), I had lost 15 pounds on your plan with no exercise or extra effort. Since then I have lost another 3 pounds and now weigh what I did when I was 25 years old. I also have more energy and do not feel deprived in any way. This is the best thing that ever happened to me. Thank you so much for giving me my life back.

You should also know that for years I suffered with digestive problems and was always running to the doctor. I was always bloated and could not digest my food for many hours and sometimes into the next day. All of these problems have disappeared as well.

As of today, my husband has lost 23 pounds, my girlfriend has lost 27 pounds, and I have several other friends and relatives who have purchased your book and started Somersizing (11 to be exact) due to my success and enthusiasm.

Thank you again and may God Bless you.

Sincerely,
Rebecca A. Vara

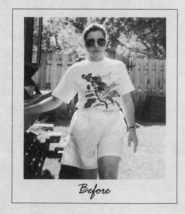

Before

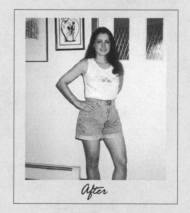

After

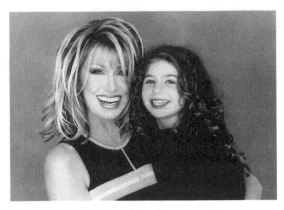

*Me and my
darling granddaughter Daisy.*

system. That's how Level Two works: you eat mostly on Level One and decide when you want to treat yourself. Sometimes I stay close to Level One with frequent but little treats here and there, like a bit of olive oil on my whole grain pasta or some wild rice in my chicken soup. Other times I stay strictly on Level One for a series of meals and then have a big treat (once a month), like a piece of birthday cake with butter cream frosting. And a few times a year I *really* treat myself and eat French fries!

Near our desert home, there is a fabulous little hamburger joint called Tyler's. Alan and I stumbled in there one day and the aroma of freshly fried potatoes almost knocked me over. What I really wanted was a hamburger with French fries and a vanilla milkshake, but I knew the bloating after the meal would not be worth the short-lived pleasure of eating it. Instead I decided it was definitely the day to call in my yearly coupon for French fries. I ordered a big plate along with a green salad. And was it ever worth it! They were hot, crispy, and

perfect. (If you're going to blow it on French fries, you should eat them alone or, better yet, with a salad. The fiber in the salad helps to diminish the effects of the fries.) Alan showed no restraint and ordered the whole shebang—hamburger, fries, and shake. As he ate, he gloated about what I was missing. Yeah, I was missing it all right . . . within an hour his system went into a tizzy from the bad combination of meat and bread on top of French fries and the bun made from white flour and the sugar in the milkshake. He wasn't much fun to be around later that day when he started burping and passing gas! Now we are regulars at Tyler's, not for the fries, but for the "Somersize burger"—a freshly grilled patty with lettuce, tomato, mayonnaise, pickle, and burned onions. Yum. No bun!

Generally I find that in Level Two I can eat a few more Carbos meals without a problem, and I can add a bit of fat. Sometimes I have whole-grain pasta or brown rice for lunch with vegetables. On Level One I have no oil with this meal, but on Level Two I can sauté the vegetables in some oil and have a more flavorful stir-fry without causing a significant imbalance. But adding protein to a Carbos meal is a little tricky. If I want to have meat with my pasta or brown rice, I would make the meal predominantly a Pro/Fats meal with a small portion of pasta or rice (maybe half a cup or so), rather than have a big bowl of pasta with a few pieces of meat. For me, the protein in combination with a significant amount of carbohydrate is harder on my body than a little fat in combination with the carbs.

If I'm going to have a sandwich, I usually

still have a vegetarian sandwich on whole-grain bread, but every now and then I add some avocado. The avocado has carbohydrate and fat in it, but as long as I don't add meat as well, I generally find I do not have a problem. I also might add a little mayonnaise or olive oil depending on the sandwich. And if I feel like having a meat or tuna fish sandwich, then I usually stick to Level One and use lettuce cups instead of bread. (If I were to eat bread with meat or tuna fish, I would use only one slice and it would definitely be whole-grain bread.)

MIXING FRUIT

I still try to eat the Fruit group completely separately. The only fruit I play around with is berries, because berries are easier to digest than other fruits. They have a very high fiber content and give me little trouble when I combine them with other foods. In Level Two I do not even think twice about eating fresh berries with whipped cream after a Pro/Fats and Veggies meal. Also, when I get tired of toast with nonfat cottage cheese or nonfat yogurt, I use a little berry jam sweetened with fruit juice, not sugar, on my toast in the morning. (Although fruit sugar and regular sugar create a similar insulin response, most fruit-sweetened jams are not as heavily sweetened as sugared jams.) And if I just have to have pancakes, I make buckwheat or whole-wheat pancakes with berry sauce instead of maple syrup. Check out my recipe for Oatmeal Pancakes with Blueberry Sauce (page 226). Regular pancakes with butter and maple syrup would create a huge imbalance, whereas whole-wheat, buckwheat, or multigrain pancakes served with berry sauce create less of an imbalance and still satisfy my craving. I also like to use berries in tarts and pies made with whole-wheat crusts—certainly not Level One fare, but easier on the system than an apple tart or a pumpkin pie. And for breakfast or a snack in the afternoon I like to have fresh berries with nonfat yogurt.

I also may add a few products that are sweetened with fruit juice. At health food stores I found a few cereals made from spelt and amaranth and kamut, flakes that are sweetened with a little fruit juice. They provide a nice change in the morning. Fruit juice, like sugar, creates an insulin response, but your body can handle a little now because your cells are not overloaded with sugar.

ADDING A LITTLE SUGAR AND FUNKY FOODS

As far as sugar goes, I loosen the reins a little. I'm not quite as diligent about hunting for sugar in sauces and salad dressings. If I'm at a restaurant, I don't worry about eating a prepared blue cheese dressing on my salad, even if it has a little sugar in it. It's not enough to cause a problem for me in Level Two as long as I'm not having any carbohydrates. I continue to avoid gravy made with white flour and very sweet sauces, like barbecue sauce. And watch out for those thick Chinese sauces made with sugar and cornstarch. Most restaurants are happy to prepare your food without these ingredients.

If I feel like having a little starch with a

Pro/Fats meal, I choose parsnips over potatoes or white rice; they're not quite as starchy. I also find I can eat moderate amounts of the foods on the Bad Combo list, such as nuts, olives, liver, avocado, and tofu.

And how about desserts? Every now and then it's okay to enjoy a dessert. On Level Two I probably eat dessert once a week; however, you may be able to eat more or less depending on your system. Some desserts aren't as bad as others. I still try to stay away from the extremely sugary ones. Take a look at the sugar content in my beloved favorite—birthday cake. Just how much sugar is in a double-layer white cake with lemon filling and butter cream frosting? Two cups of sugar in the cake, half a cup in the lemon filling, plus one more cup in the frosting. Three and a half cups of sugar! Add the copious amounts of white flour, which are a Funky Food, and the butter and eggs (Pro/Fats), and you have a poorly combined Pro/Fat, Carbo, Funky Food concoction sure to send your system into mayhem.

Check out some of my recipes for low-sugar desserts. My Strawberry Gratin is made from berries, sour cream, and a touch of brown sugar: a much better option for Somersizing purposes. But the beauty of this program is that if you really want it, you can have white cake with lemon filling and butter cream frosting—you'll just have to live back on Level One for longer.

Another good dessert option after a Pro/Fat meal is a piece of cheesecake with fresh berries. Cheesecake is often lower in sugar than other desserts and is made mostly of Pro/Fats: eggs, cream cheese, sour cream, and lemon juice. Pudding, crème brûlée, chocolate mousse, and even ice cream are generally lower in sugar than most other desserts, and they do not have the addition of white flour as many other pastries do. And as I mentioned, flourless chocolate cake is a great option in Level Two, as are strawberries dipped in chocolate with freshly whipped cream!

You really can eat these desserts and maintain your weight if you are Somersizing properly. Check out my recipes for Level Two desserts. You'll be knocked out by how great they are. They are all relatively low in sugar, and I use whole-wheat pastry flour instead of white flour. I have included a few desserts made with artificial sweetener that can be eaten occasionally on Level One. Although technically these artificially sweetened desserts are Level One fare, I don't want you eating chemically laden desserts after every meal and thinking they are perfectly okay since they have no sugar. I have included them so that you have an alternative to a sugary dessert on special occasions while you are diligently sticking to your Level One guidelines. As my son-in-law, Frank (my personal trainer), said to me, "You should not make diet desserts. Desserts are not diet food. Eat real desserts, but not too often." He's absolutely right.

YOU'RE IN CONTROL

As far as Level Two goes, you are in control. Maybe you don't miss the sweets as much as you miss the bread. Then save your treats for a great baguette or a chewy sourdough roll. Or if it's white pasta you're craving, eat mostly Level One meals and then indulge yourself with a little pasta fix. It's up to you. For me, the whole-grain pasta is so good that I don't ever feel deprived eating it instead of white pasta. Sometimes I even bring it to my favorite Italian restaurants and ask the kitchen to use it instead of white pasta. They never seem to mind, as long as I pay full price for my dish. I still stay away from meat sauce with my whole-grain pasta because the combination makes me bloat.

The other night Alan and I stopped by our favorite little Tuscan restaurant for dinner. They have the best Italian food, a real Italian chef, and real Italian waiters. I started with an arugula and radicchio salad with shaved Parmesan cheese. For dinner I ordered the Tuscan pounded steak with rosemary and garlic. It came with sautéed spinach and roasted potatoes (I substituted the spuds for more spinach). So far I'm still on Level One. I dipped into Level Two when I ordered a glass of red wine. And after dinner I enjoyed a small scoop of their amazing homemade coconut ice cream. Since I stuck to Level One for most of the meal, I treated myself with wine and ice cream. Alan really wanted the special, which was homemade asparagus ravioli. He also had the same salad and a glass of wine. His was predominantly a Carbos and Veggies meal, but he did have some Pro/Fats (some oil in the salad dressing and the pasta sauce and Parmesan cheese on the salad and the pasta). After this meal he did not order a dessert, because he'd used up his imbalances on the white pasta and the addition of the oil, cheese, and wine. We both had fabulous meals, and we each had to give up only a little something while still feeling indulged.

How you choose your imbalances depends on several factors. How many imbalances have you had today, and how big were your imbalances today? How many big imbalances have you had this week? Don't get cocky with your new figure! The pounds can creep their way back onto your body if you're not careful. This summer when Alan and I were in France, I made exactly that mistake. Since I was quite thin before we left (five pounds below my average weight), I decided to indulge myself around every corner. Wine with lunch? Well, I'm on vacation, I would think. A piece of baguette with your Brie? Well, I'm on vacation. A lovely French tart with your cappuccino? Why not . . . I'm on vacation. Day after day as we strolled though Paris I continued with a little sugar here, some Funky Foods there, and bad combinations. Before I knew it I was eating as though I had no knowledge of Somersizing. And I should know better!

One morning we slept quite late (jet lag). We had missed breakfast, but I was so tired I ordered a regular cappuccino and a glass of orange juice. I sat on the charming terrace overlooking the city and sipped my coffee and orange juice. Wow, did my heart start pounding! As I was doing it, I was wondering why I was drinking caffeine when I know the ill effects it has on my body. By the time we got showered, dressed, and out of the hotel it was after one-thirty and all the restaurants were closed for lunch. The only thing we could find open was a *crêperie*. Oh well, I convinced myself, I'm on vacation.

Alan and I both ordered crepes for lunch. The thin, delicate French pancakes were filled with spinach, mushrooms, and cheese. Delicious. I requested the crepes made with buckwheat flour, so the overall effect wasn't that bad. But afterward those dessert crepes were staring me in the face, and I thought, Well, I'm on vacation. The dessert crepes were made the traditional way, with white flour, milk, and butter, then cooked, filled with preserves, and topped with powdered sugar. Sugar overload! The pleasure was fleeting at best. Within twenty minutes I had a stomachache so bad that I thought I was having an attack of appendicitis. Alan suggested we take a walk and try to shake it off. I was uncomfortable and irritable. Every suggestion he made seemed like a stupid one. Reluctantly I agreed to the walk. But after my sugar high, I dipped so low that I couldn't walk anymore, and I turned on Alan! We started to argue (over nothing), and we never argue. I told him I had to go back to the hotel and have a nap.

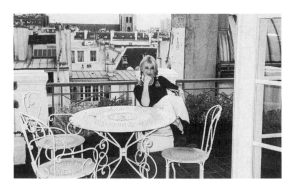

Me, mad and upset, sitting on our hotel terrace in Paris after having a sugar binge—it wasn't worth it.

As we made our way back we argued more, and I told him I never wanted to come to Paris again. Back in the hotel he promptly fell asleep while I sat on my beautiful terrace and cried for two hours, hoping he'd hear me and ask what was wrong. What *was* wrong? I had no idea . . . but I was an absolute wreck! Finally I cried myself to sleep and ended the ugly episode.

Of all people, you would think I should know better! A caffeine, sugar, and white flour overload threw my system into chaos and ruined what could have been a perfectly lovely day in Paris. Instead I was physically racked and an emotional wreck from making bad food choices. It was no treat to eat crepes.

Ironically, that same week my daughter-in-law, Caroline, called me in Paris to tell me she had a great Somersizing story to tell me.

Bruce, Caroline, and their daughters, Camelia and Violet, were vacationing at our beach house in Los Angeles with their friends Sydelle, Siavash, and their two little girls. On Sunday morning Camelia requested French pancakes, just as her cousin Ziane eats. Ziane is our grandchild who lives in France with our son Stephen and his beautiful wife, Olivia. Caroline pulled out the flour and the milk and the butter and lovingly made crepes for everyone but herself. She was still trying to lose the last bit of weight from her pregnancy and was following Level One guidelines. The little girls covered their hot crepes in butter and jam. Sydelle ate hers with butter, lemon juice, and powdered sugar. Siavash went for the butter and syrup, and Bruce ate his first few batches with butter, syrup, and powdered sugar, then switched to butter, lemon juice, and powdered sugar and ended back with the syrup! "I'm going for it," Bruce bragged, "'cause I'm on vacation!" (The apple doesn't fall far from the tree.) After everyone had eaten, Caroline cooked five slices of bacon until they were crisp and then fried two eggs in the bacon drippings for herself.

As they ate they talked about what they wanted to do for the rest of the day. Caroline and Sydelle wanted to go shopping for antiques. The little girls talked excitedly about taking a walk down to the shore with their dads to play in the ocean. Bruce and Siavash made reservations at nearby courts to play racquetball. But within an hour the effects of the crepes had set in. Caroline said she looked around and was astonished at how the sugar and white flour had knocked everyone down like dominos. The children were cranky and started fighting with one another, too tired to walk to the shore. Sydelle was asking Bruce to make some strong coffee because she needed a caffeine fix. Bruce wanted to help her, but he was slumped over in a chair, looking as though he had an incredible hangover. He looked at Caroline and said, "Wow. I can't eat sugar anymore. I feel like I've been punched." And where was Siavash? He'd retreated to his room for a midmorning nap! So much for shopping, swimming, or racquetball . . . the only one who had energy to do anything was the ol' bacon-and-eggs girl, Caroline! She said she felt as if she'd poisoned her family and friends with those delicious but deadly crepes.

So beware of the slipups. It usually starts with one dessert, which leads to another and then another. Before you know it, you've started adding bad combinations and a little white flour here and there. Your body will alert you with warning signs. Learn to listen to them! If you start craving sugar and carbohydrates, it means you are eating too many of them. That's what happens; the more sugar you eat, the more you crave. Then come the energy dips, the extra pounds, and don't forget about the damage you're doing on the inside to your healthy cells. Remember, the best way to take away a sugar craving is to eat a Pro/Fat because Pro/Fats help to stabilize blood sugar. So next time you have a craving for sugar or carbohydrates, eat a piece of cheese and it should help the problem. All in all, if you notice signs that your body is starting to crave sugar again, go back to Level One until you get rid of the problem. Stay on top of the new you. Take care of your body.

I also want to mention a few words about portion control. On Level One you may eat as much as you want as long as you are following *all* the Level One guidelines. (That means technically you can gorge yourself and not gain weight, although I'm sure you will not end up overeating, because your appetite will be fully satisfied with wholesome, nutritious foods.) In Level Two you must consider limiting your portions when you are creating imbalances. You can't have it both ways—the bonus of Level One is that you can eat as much as you want. The bonus of Level Two is that you have more variety, but you must limit your portions moderately.

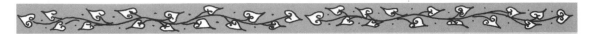

A SOMERSIZING SUCCESS STORY

Dear Suzanne,

I bought your book *Eat Great, Lose Weight*. The Sunday after Easter, April 13, I started your diet. It changed my life. In about 12 weeks I lost 25 pounds! I plan to eat this way the rest of my life. It is fun and I eat better than I ever did in my life; and now for the first time, I enjoy eating.

I really didn't need to lose much weight, but my stomach was the problem. No matter how much exercise I did, my stomach wouldn't go down flat until after I started your diet. Now my stomach is flat. I'm not bloated and I don't have gas.

Your diet really works! Even now when I go out for the day, I still take my food and fruit with me so I can Somersize. I look good and I feel good; better than I ever did, and I have lots of energy. Everywhere I go people tell me how good I look.

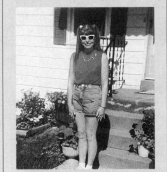

I feel so good and so happy now. Thank you for sharing your book and diet with us.

A fan of yours,
Regina Berres

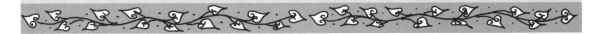

WINE AND CHOCOLATE

Part of the variety of Level Two includes wine and chocolate. Recently studies have shown that red wine has been proven to have beneficial effects on the heart by helping to keep arteries clear. I have incorporated it, in moderation, in Level Two. A glass or two of wine with your meals is perfectly fine. I use wine freely in many of my recipes in Level One and Two. It creates only a slight imbalance because most of the alcohol is cooked off in the process. It wonderfully enhances the flavor of my meals and does not seem to disrupt my system. If you are progressing well on Level One, you should not have a problem doing the same.

Now for chocolate . . . my great love! In fact, if I had to choose between chocolate and Alan . . . well, I'd choose Alan, but it wouldn't be easy! I can't seem to live without chocolate; and I don't have to. Dark chocolate (more than 60 percent cocoa) is relatively low in sugar and does not create a huge imbalance. The best time to eat chocolate is on an empty stomach, perhaps a couple of squares in the afternoon. And I have many sinful low-sugar desserts made from dark chocolate that are perfect for Level Two.

You will continue to use all of the recipes in Level One for Level Two. In addition, I have included a few recipes specific to Level Two for your enjoyment. Good luck in this new phase. You have such freedom in Level Two, I just know you will love it. Any questions you have will be answered by your own body as you experi-ment. Eating this way is truly a pleasure, and I'm sure you will be the envy of all of your friends, who won't believe what wonderful foods you eat and still manage to keep your beautiful figure.

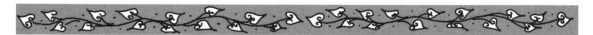

A SOMERSIZING SUCCESS STORY

Dear Suzanne,

I am a practicing gynecologist in Chattanooga, Tennessee. Over the years my patients have tried many different diets, most of which eventually failed. They usually ended up weighing more than when they started. After talking to them about dieting I found that most of them felt deprived when dieting. They were able to get themselves psyched up for a short period of time, but were unable to maintain the extreme discipline, focus, and motivation necessary for a lifetime change.

As I grew older, I became 23 pounds overweight myself. Like my patients, I tried all the diet plans, to no avail. Then one day my daughter-in-law sent my wife your *Eat Great, Lose Weight*. My wife asked me to try it with her, and, reluctantly, I agreed, explaining to her that all diets are the same and the end result is failure. Boy! Was I ever wrong! In March 1997 I started to Somersize and in three months I lost 23 pounds and reached my goal. Needless to say, I feel much better physically and have much more energy with the extra weight off.

I had such great success personally, I have placed my patients on your Somersize program and recommended it to my friends. I am thoroughly convinced it is the way to go.

Sincerely yours,
Stanley J. Dressler, M.D.

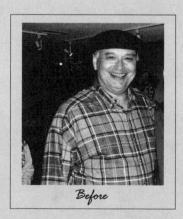

Before

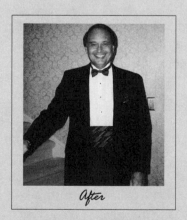

After

ELEVEN

Why We Eat

So often we find ourselves staring into the refrigerator thinking, What can I eat? What can I eat? We ask ourselves this question not always because we are physically hungry for food, but rather because we need to fill some emotional void that is begging for attention. It seems easier to fill that void by eating foods that our bodies do not need or want.

Didn't get that job you were pitching for? Go out and grab a hamburger with some friends. Depressed over your love life . . . or lack thereof? Snuggle up with a gallon of ice cream and a squirt bottle full of chocolate sauce. Feeling lonely? Down a bag of cheese puffs and Snowballs. Family problems too big to deal with? Have some macaroni and cheese. Sound familiar? Almost all of us have used food at certain times in our lives to act as a friend or lover or to fill some emotional need that we'd rather not face. It doesn't matter if we are hungry or full; food

becomes the great distractor, a vice that helps us put off the inevitable feelings we all have to face.

This type of overeating ranges from the occasional munchie session to the serious compulsive overeating problem that plagues thousands and thousands of people across the globe. Eating disorders run rampant among young women, pulling one after the next into the dark world of bulimia and anorexia. Professional health care workers almost all agree across the board that addictions to food stem from emotional problems. Control issues often surface when we discuss unhealthy patterns with food.

What in your life has you feeling out of control? Do you have issues you refuse to face? What pain are you hiding from that keeps you from living the happy, healthy balanced life you long for? Do you use food as a numbing device to keep you from feeling the pain deep inside?

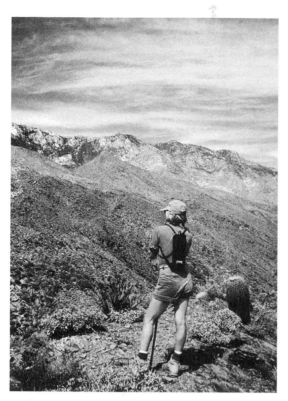

Hiking is not only a physical experience but a spiritual one as well.

Many of us use different devices to numb the pain in our lives. Some do it with alcohol, like my father. Some do it with drugs or sex. Personally, I did it with shopping. When I was a young woman in my twenties, I would buy things I couldn't afford. It was part of a fantasy life I created for myself and those around me. Growing up with an alcoholic left me with a self-esteem so damaged, I felt I needed to create a different person—a person I thought others would like. Unlike the real me, *she* could afford nice things and *she* came from a perfect family with plenty of money. Living this lie got me into a load of trouble. I was even

arrested for writing bad checks. Even worse, I jeopardized my relationship with Alan by lying to him for years about my real family.

It wasn't until I did "the work" with a therapist that I was able to unravel the pain of my past and get on with the life I wanted to lead. Doing the work was long and hard. It was agitating because it stirred up uncomfortable old feelings I didn't want to go back and face. However uncomfortable, facing that pain in my life allowed me to find resolution so I could move forward spiritually and emotionally. Slowly I began to build my self-worth and was able to begin the life I finally felt I deserved. It was not until then that things fell into place for me. I got the relationship I wanted with Alan. I began the career I longed for as an actress and I was able to begin the fulfilling life I had dreamed about as a little girl.

You can have this, too. You probably picked up this book because you would like to find your ideal body weight. In order to get the body you want, you first have to get your head in order. If you skip that crucial step, you may have a hard time committing to this or any program designed to promote health. Even if you commit to the food guidelines, you must get your head in order if you want to keep the weight off for good; otherwise, when you have an emotional slip, your bad eating habits will follow.

So next time you find yourself alone with only the glow of the refrigerator light staring you in the face, ask yourself, Am I really hungry or am I eating to fill some other void? Am I eating to put off some other task I should be handling? Am I eating because I am depressed or because I had a fight with my spouse, or because I have pain buried so deep inside that I'm just not ready to face? I urge you to deal with your unresolved emotions that keep you emotionally and physically handicapped. The first step is closing the refrigerator door, unless you can honestly say that you are eating because your body is sending you hunger signals for a nutritious meal. You can have the life you've always dreamed of. It is waiting for you to find it. I know, because I have been there. I wish you the best of luck.

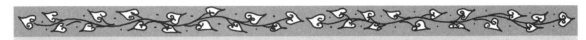

A SOMERSIZING SUCCESS STORY

Dear Suzanne,

I wanted to let you know that your book *Eat Great, Lose Weight* has helped me to lose 38 pounds that I have needed to lose for a long time.

I will be 50 this summer and as an adult have always struggled with my weight. I have been successful in losing weight at least 4 times but have always gained it back eventually. My primary motivation has always been to look better—not because it was the healthy thing to do.

Last summer when I went in for a long-overdue physical, I was told that I had high blood pressure and cholesterol. My genes were finally catching up with me. My father died of a heart attack at 55 and I knew that I needed to do something.

In February I saw you on the Home Shopping Club talking about your book. I am by nature cautious and did not buy your book that day but did go to a bookstore to look it over. I did that a couple of times before I finally purchased it.

I guess your program just hit me at the right time because I started the day after I got it, February 9, and lost 35 pounds by June 15. It had been increasingly difficult for me to lose weight as I grew older so I never expected this kind of result. I am now at a weight that I believe is good for me. I don't weigh what I did at 20 but my doctor is happy and I can wear a size 10 or 12.

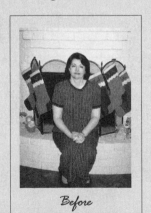

Before

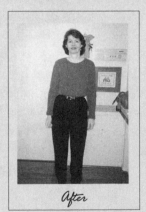

After

I am now ready for Level 2. I am a little apprehensive I must admit. I don't want to repeat past behavior and start putting the weight on again but I am optimistic that this time will be different.

Thanks again.
Sincerely,
Lynn Peterson

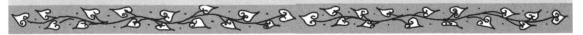

Part Two

COOKING—

IT'S A FAMILY

AFFAIR!

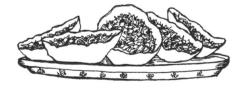

TWELVE

Family Dinners

One of the great joys of my life is cooking wonderful food for my family. Conversations with all of us sitting around the dinner table are my most treasured times. As a child, my mother tried to make home-cooked meals for us whenever she could, and I always loved to help her with the preparation. One Christmas I was given a *real* electric child's stove. It was the equivalent of a hot burner (child safety laws would never allow it today), but it looked exactly like a grown-up stove. I loved it. There were packages of cake mix, and I baked and frosted my first cakes at six years old. This probably started my love affair with cake. I also had a real porcelain miniature tea set with six cups and saucers, creamer, sugar bowl, and six plates. I would set up my little table made from an orange crate covered with a tablecloth from my mother's collection of embroidered linens. I'd pick baby rosebuds from a bush in our garden and

make darling little nosegay bouquets to complete my setting. A hostess in training was born.

I developed my love for cooking at this time, and my mother encouraged that side of me, praising me endlessly. Her support of my interest in food and its presentation was vitally important to my development. Because of my father's alcoholism, the dinners my mother put out were often disrupted. Things would become tense and uncomfortable, sometimes even violent. But not all the memories are tainted. There were lots of laughs and joking around with my brothers and sister. And when I went out and started a family of my own, I wanted to be sure that mealtimes were safe and nurturing, so I took the opportunity to create the tradition of family dinners.

Dinner is a time to turn off the television and connect as a family. Everyone has been out during the day, taking care of business.

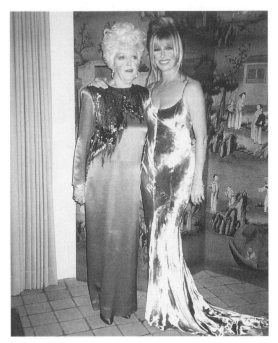

*My beautiful mother and me, ready for
a night on the town.*

Dinnertime provides the opportunity to check in with the ones you love and find out what's going on in their lives. If all the family members are transfixed by the television, deep, meaningful conversation is virtually impossible. In order to connect, you must take the time to focus on one another. "How was your day?" may sound like a trivial question, but it can become the beginning of a meaningful conversation if you're ready to share and listen.

I've always felt that children, especially, need the structure of family dinners on a regular basis. It's easy to fragment into your separate bedrooms to get homework done or talk on the phone, but it is up to parents to make dinner a mandatory event. If it's a

ritual started from youth, the family looks forward to it. Bruce and I have had our best talks while eating home-cooked meals together. When he was a little boy I was a single mother, and even though it was just the two of us, we usually sat down together and ate as a family. He's always loved my cooking. Most kids request macaroni and cheese or pizza, but Bruce's favorites were steamed clams with garlic butter or home-made chicken soup. I have great pride knowing I raised him on healthy, delicious, nutritious foods that he loved. I never had to force him to finish anything . . . he gobbled up my meals with joy.

We're all busy, and sometimes family dinner is simply not possible, but I make that case an exception to the rule. I make ordering "takeout" a rarity. Everyone is busy and time is a premium, but preparing meals for your family need not take any more than thirty minutes. (Most of the recipes mentioned in the following meal plans can be found in this book. The others are listed in *Eat Great, Lose Weight*.) Many of the recipes in this book can be prepared in that amount of time or less. All it takes is a little organization and the willingness to make it a priority. Wash a few heads of lettuce on Sunday and store them in plastic bags so making your green salad is a snap. Keep plenty of meat, poultry, and seafood in the freezer and defrost a package by placing it in the refrigerator before you go to bed at night. It will be ready for the following night's dinner. Then all you have to do to create a great dinner is wash and chop some vegetables—maybe some broccoli and cauliflower to throw in the steamer. Brown an onion and some garlic in olive oil. Season the meat with salt, pepper, and your favorite herb, then pan-fry it. Remove the meat when cooked and add some broth or wine to the pan and scrape up the brown bits that have accumulated on the bottom of the pan to make a fabulous sauce. (It also makes cleanup a breeze because you're cleaning the cooked parts off the bottom of the pan!) Turn off the heat, add a pat of butter, and pour the sauce over the meat and vegetables. Toss your salad with a little olive oil and lemon juice and you're ready to sit down.

And don't forget how fast, easy, and delicious meals can be prepared on the barbecue. Prep your meat in advance by marinating it for a couple of hours or even overnight. Or if you don't have time, just coat it with some olive oil, salt, and pepper and throw it on the grill. Slice your vegetables, brush them lightly with olive oil, and toss them on, too. Try zucchini, yellow squash, mushrooms, fennel, peppers, tomatoes, eggplant, and more. The only thing greater than the flavor is the fact that there are no pots and pans to clean!

Remember to make the whole family a part of the preparation and cleanup process. If Mom does the washing and chopping, maybe Dad does the grilling while the kids set the table. And everyone helps clean up. When it's dinnertime, it's family time. If it's not a ritual in your house, make it one. You won't believe what you're missing.

Today Alan and I have the combined family we have always dreamed of. All of our children are grown and married, with children of their own. We now have four grandchildren. How blessed we are! On the following pages you'll get a glimpse of what family dinners are like at our home. Some of the meals are quite fancy, while others are seemingly uneventful and simple. But at each meal there is a connection—a connection to the people I love the most in this world. And I am grateful for every opportunity to gather round a table to share food, laughter, and love with the beautiful people I call "family."

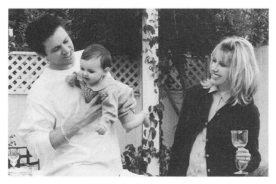

Bruce loves being a father.

A Winter Pork Roast in Palm Springs

Twelve-Hour Roast Pork (page 222)

Parsnip Puree with Roasted Garlic (page 234)

Shredded Brussels Sprouts with Lime Juice (EGLW, page 99)

Fire-Roasted Cherry Peppers

Cappuccino Chocolate Chunk Cheesecake (page 246)

Nothing hits the spot in winter like a pork roast. In January we often found ourselves at our desert home, rejuvenating our souls from the hustle and bustle of Los Angeles. Leslie, Frank, and Daisy joined us for the weekend. I spent hours in the pool with Daisy as she jumped time and again into my arms from the side of the pool. All the while we could smell the succulent scents wafting from the kitchen fans. Then Alan would take Daisy for a ride in the golf cart down to the new playground we built at the bottom of the property.

In the afternoon we all retreated to our rooms for a rest and reconvened at dinner as a family. On those long, slow days in the desert I love to make my 12-hour pork roast shoulder. It slow-cooks for a whole day so that the outside gets a wonderful crispy texture from the frequent drizzling of freshly squeezed lemon juice over the top. The lemon and the addition of cayenne pepper make this meal a winner. I served it with parsnip and roasted garlic puree, Brussels sprouts with a kick of lime juice, and fire-roasted cherry peppers brushed with olive oil and thrown on the grill to liven up the plate. As we devoured the crispy, succulent pork, one would never imagine we were losing weight, but most of the meal followed Level One guidelines. Only the parsnips and the dessert, my cappuccino chocolate cheesecake, created a minor imbalance. Since we were all cruising along in Level Two, we ate without guilt.

FEBRUARY

A Drop-by at Bruce and Caroline's

*Milanese Beef with Sautéed Onions and Mushrooms
in a Port Wine Sauce (page 208)*

Steamed Broccoli

*Endive and Radicchio Salad with Stilton Cheese
and Balsamic Vinaigrette (page 141)*

Easy Ice Cream Coffee Treat (page 251)

Bruce and Caroline live only five minutes away from us in their darling Santa Monica home. We love being able to drop by and say hello to them on our way home. I always call first!

Nothing gives parents more pride than seeing their children happy. When I see the happiness that Bruce has achieved in his life, I simply want to burst! He and Caroline have built a wonderful life together. Four years ago they bought the ugliest house on their street, and since then they have fixed it up to be this little cottage that oozes with charm. They have formed their own production company, which has become so successful that they are winning accounts over the biggest ad agencies in the country. And they have given life to two of our adorable grandchildren, Camelia and Violet. (Yes, all three of my granddaughters are flower girls.)

Last February, on one of our drop-bys, we found Caroline, Bruce, and Camelia preparing a wonderful dinner. Caroline was about eight months pregnant with Violet at the time. They insisted they had enough for all of us and asked us to stay for dinner. I didn't want to impose, but if you'd seen what they were making, you would have stayed, too! Caroline had been marinating Milanese beef, a thinly pounded sirloin, for several hours in port wine, olive oil, garlic, soy sauce, and lemon juice. After Camelia helped pull the stems off the mushrooms, Caroline chopped them and cooked them down with caramelized onions. When the mushrooms were crusty, she deglazed the pan with port and scraped the bits off the bottom of the pan. "Zannie [that's me] taught me how to make the best sauce just by using the bits on the bottom of the pan," Caroline told Camelia. "And now I'm going to teach you how to do it, too." After the mushrooms and onions were finished, Caroline removed them from the pan and quickly seared the steaks on each side. The final step was to deglaze the pan again with port to capture the flavor of the meat. She let the sauce reduce, then turned off the heat and added a little butter to richen the flavor.

Bruce made one of his incredible salads with radicchio, endive, and Stilton cheese.

Then he let Camelia toss it with the olive oil and balsamic vinegar. Camelia's only two, and already she loves to help cook! When the broccoli was steamed, we were ready to eat. Incredible flavors, and the meat was so tender that you could cut it with your fork. Only the dessert threw us into Level Two. Bruce pulled out a carton of Häagen-Dazs vanilla ice cream and poured hot decaf coffee over the top, which makes a little frosty crust on the ice cream. Simple and delicious.

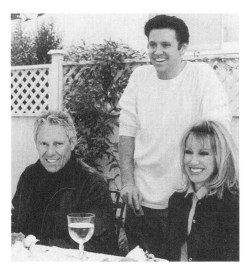

Me with my two favorite men — Alan, my husband, and Bruce, my son.

Leg of Lamb by the Sea

Marinated Grilled Butterflied Leg of Lamb (page 219)

Baked Caramelized Onions (page 179)

Steamed Asparagus

Chopped Raw Zucchini
and Parmesan Salad (page 143)

Almond Chocolate Torte with Whipped Cream (page 247)

Spring is the season for lamb. If I had to choose a favorite meat, it would be lamb. It has the most incredible flavor, especially when you slather it with olive oil, loads of garlic, and fresh rosemary. In March we had a Sunday night dinner on the roof of our beach house while Alan's sister, Cissy, and her husband Lewis were in town. Plus, Stephen, Leslie, Frank, Daisy, Bruce, Caroline, Camelia, and Violet came over. For me, Sunday dinners are the perfect time to make something special for my family. During the week I'm so rushed, I don't have time to prepare elaborate meals. But on Sundays there is nothing that brings me more pleasure.

In the morning I prepped the lamb. I pierced it all over, then covered it with olive oil, garlic, fresh rosemary, sea salt, and cracked black pepper. I set that aside in the refrigerator to marinate and began on my dessert: a fabulous chocolate nut torte. It has no added sugar (only the sugar in the dark chocolate) and is mixed with ground nuts, eggs, and butter. It's a perfect Level Two dessert, only a minor imbalance and well worth it.

Alan and I took a bike ride on the strand in the afternoon. We have a tandem bike, and riding up the coast is one of our favorite ways to connect and get some exercise at the same time. And the great thing about a tandem bike is that it's really easy to hear one another talking, unlike riding side by side yelling all the while.

When we got home, Alan started heating the grill to get it good and hot. After about an hour he threw the butterflied leg of lamb on the hot grill to sear it on both sides, sealing in the juices. Meanwhile I was in the kitchen, preparing the red onions (my favorite part of the dinner). You score the onion and shove a few cloves of garlic in the middle along with some butter, fresh thyme, salt, and pepper. Then I placed them side by side in a roasting pan, poured balsamic vinegar and red wine over the top, and baked them for two hours until they became these incredible caramelized pink rosettes with a wonderful reduction of balsamic vinegar and wine to spoon over the top.

Everyone flipped over the dinner. The lamb was perfect. Alan is the ultimate grill master. And the flavor of the onions was to die for! Even the little girls gobbled them up. We had delicious, fresh spring vegetables and a salad of arugula with raw zucchini, olive oil, fresh lemon juice, salt, pepper, and shaved Parmesan cheese. Would you ever guess we were losing weight? Then I pulled out the chocolate nut torte and sat quietly as the table echoed with "yummy noises." Okay, so after the torte we were no longer losing weight, but we were well within Level Two to maintain our weight. And if you basically follow Level One during the week, a dessert on Sunday is an acceptable imbalance. That's what I love about Somersizing: it allows you to enjoy mealtimes without feeling deprived.

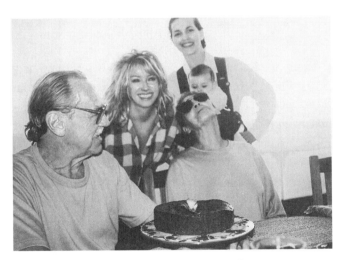

My famous Chocolate Almond Torte served on the rooftop with my brother-in-law Lewis and sister-in-law Cecile, me, Caroline, and Violet.

APRIL

Violet's Christening

Lamb Skewers with Harissa Dipping Sauce (page 218)

Hummus with Whole-Wheat Pita Bread (EGLW, page 77)

Hearts of Palm Salad (page 147)

*Garden Greens with Pear Tomatoes
and Lemon-Mint Vinaigrette (page 139)*

Crudités with Roasted Vegetable Dip (page 153)

Roasted Vegetable Sandwiches (page 231)

*Penne Pasta with Green Beans
and Feta Cheese (page 232)*

Dessert Assortment

Our fourth grandchild was born in April . . . our sweet little Violet. I bonded with her instantly. I call her the "I don't want to be a bother" baby because she is so good-natured. From the start she was a good sleeper, and she rarely has fussy periods. What a wonderful addition to the family.

Her birth was particularly special to me because it came just weeks after my mother's sudden passing. Violet's christening was held at Bruce and Caroline's parish, where they were married seven years ago. My mother was a devout Catholic, and I thought of her frequently as the priest welcomed this tiny baby into the church. Violet stared attentively at the priest as he blessed her and anointed her head with oil. And she didn't even make a peep when he poured the water over her head.

After the lovely ceremony we had the entire family over for a celebration at our home. In honor of the tiny "guest of honor," I covered our dining room table with small potted violets and freshly cut magnolias. The platters of bountiful food gave plenty of options for a Level One Pro/Fats and Veggies

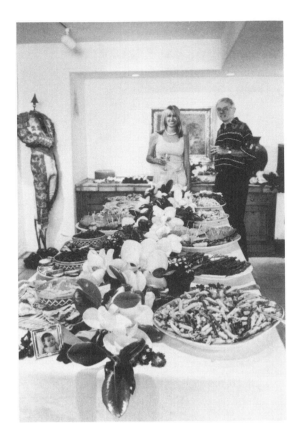

Violet's christening feast (see the small picture of her on the left).

I always try to prepare food for my guests myself, but on certain occasions, such as Violet's Christening Day, we all need a little help; that's when I call my friend Ken Brown. Ken is a fabulous chef who recently opened a storefront in West Hollywood called Urban Epicuria. When Ken describes his business, he says, "We specialize in gourmet take-away." When I describe it I say he specializes in excellence. His food is fresh and packed with flavor. It can be heated to perfection without getting soggy, tough, or overcooked. Ken's a lifesaver, especially when you have fifty people coming to your home who will be arriving at the same time you are! He was even generous enough to share a few of his fabulous recipes, which you'll find later in the book.

The day was perfect yet bittersweet. It marked the first family function since my mother's death, and her absence left a hole in my heart. We were extremely close, and I miss her dearly. When you have a great mother, as I did, you sometimes feel she is the only person in the whole world who truly understands you. That bond, that connection, that trust, cannot be replaced. Yet the cycle of life continues. Now we are gifted with a baby, a perfectly healthy, beautiful baby girl who has eyes to match the color of her name and a soul that seems to mimic the gentleness of her great-grandmother.

meal, or for a Level Two meal if you added the Carbos dishes. The food tasted fresh and delicious, and little Violet had a great day—soaking up all the incredible energy from the surrounding family and friends who already love her so deeply.

Father's Day and Birthday Celebration at Leslie and Frank's

Greek Salad (EGLW, page 113)

Frank's Amazing Chicken (Lemon Roasted Chicken)
(EGLW, page 158)

Cheesecake Bar (page 246)

Leslie and Frank throw fabulous dinner parties. We always look forward to eating at their home. This year we celebrated Alan's birthday and Father's Day on the same day because we were going to be out of town on his actual birthday. I love going to Leslie and Frank's home to see how Leslie's creativity has manifested itself. She is an incredible artist. Last time we went to dinner she had covered her enormous living room with a leopard-print rug—and it looks fabulous! Recently she decided to give the dining room a face-lift, and she had the walls painted Pepto-Bismol pink with alternating orange and gold trim hand-painted on the baroque moldings. It looks like an exotic butterfly.

Leslie is an amazing designer; in fact, she designs all my saucy little outfits for *Candid Camera*. She has an eye for beautiful fabric and sleek lines. I can't tell you how many

cards and letters I've received from people telling me how much they love my clothes on the show! She's quite a talent. There is no one I would rather have designing for me than Leslie.

Both Leslie and Frank excel in the kitchen; they're excellent cooks. He's a bodybuilder (former Mr. France), a personal trainer, a master of krau magá (an Israeli form of self-defense), and an action hero in training. With that face and that body, watch out, Jean-Claude Van Damme! But of all his talents, it is his chicken I revere him for most. Frank makes the best baked chicken I've ever had. The outside gets a wonderful crusty texture, while the inside stays moist and delicious. And he puts on a ton of seasoning, like cayenne, herbs, lemon juice, salt, and pepper. To go with the chicken, Leslie made a Greek salad with tomatoes, red onion, feta cheese, cucumber, and kalamata olives. It was a divine combination. Simple foods, the freshest ingredients, and perfect preparation.

Caroline and Bruce brought Alan's birthday cake—two cheesecakes, one made with sugar and the other made with artificial sweetener. They also brought three different sauces to choose from: chocolate ganache, raspberry sauce, and caramel sauce. To sprinkle over the top they had fresh berries, chunks of fresh mango, or dark chocolate shavings. Everyone designed their own cheesecake creation with either the Level One sugarless cheesecake or the Level Two Choices, with varying levels of imbalance depending on how much sugar you added in the sauce and on top. I ate mine plain, because I love the simple taste of great cheesecake.

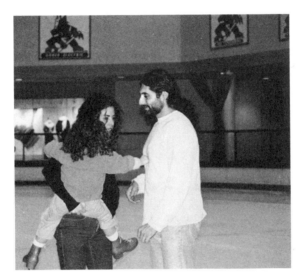

Leslie, Frank, and our granddaughter Daisy.

JUNE
A Little Lunch at the Château

Farm-Raised Chicken St. Germain Beaupré (page 195)

Mushroom Farci (page 165)

Steamed Haricots Verts

Lamb's Lettuce Salad with Warmed Goat Cheese (page 138)

Ginger Crème Brûlée (page 241)

In June we took our annual trip to France to see Alan's son Stephen, his wife, Olivia, and our grandson Ziane. They live near the Luxembourg Gardens in Paris in the most fabulous apartment. It's one of the old bourgeoisie apartments with five fabulous arched windows and twelve-foot-high ceilings. Your status in Paris is often determined by the number of windows in your apartment—and five is an impressive number. They don't care about the status, of course, they just like the view. While they were fixing up the place, they removed some paint off a wall in preparation to repaint—but underneath they found original frescoes from the turn of the century!

I guess great housing runs in the family. Olivia's father, Jean Pierre (who was the first person to teach me about food combining), recently bought a château in cen-

tral France. Yes, a château, complete with moat, electric drawbridge, fourteen bedrooms, and fourteen bathrooms on fifty-six acres of forest with two lakes! We went down to visit for the weekend and stayed in what used to be the king's room. I, of course, come from a long line of maids, so I felt very comfortable *making* the bed in the king's room. The ceilings must have been fifteen feet high, with walls eight feet thick. Stephen took me and Ziane fishing in the lake. Alan yelled to us, "What are you using for bait?" "Camembert," Stephen replied. How poetic.

One night for dinner I cooked a meal fit for a king. We shopped in the village and picked up a farm-raised chicken. I prepared it with a technique I learned from Olivia's mother, Mizou. I have learned so much from her about cooking. I boiled the chicken in a pot for about twenty minutes, then roasted it on very high heat for another twenty minutes or so. The result? It was brown and crisp on the outside, moist and tender inside. And because we happened to be in the height of mushroom season, I made a farci of mushrooms, shallots, and thyme, then cooked it down with wine and at the end stirred in a pat of butter. Plus we had a delicate salad of field greens with warmed goat cheese and steamed haricots verts (baby string beans).

For the Level Two crowd, Jean Pierre opened an incredible bottle of Rothschild to round out the meal perfectly. For dessert I made a rich and creamy raspberry crème brûlée. When in France . . . eat like the French! Even though it created a slight imbalance, it was worth it. That's the beauty of this program. You can take part in the entire experience of the food and the surroundings. The table was set in the grand dining salon of the château, and we lit the room with candles, just as it would have been done in the eleventh century when the castle was built. The French windows were hung with heavy velvet, and the stone walls dripped with ancient tapestries. It was a walk back in time, a magical meal in a magical room.

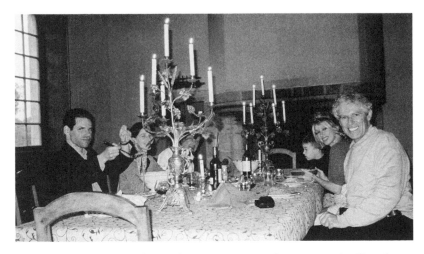

Dinner at Jean Pierre's château in France with Stephen, Olivia, Ziane, Alan and me—we are eating chicken St. Germain Beaupré.

J U L Y

Fourth of July at the Beach with a Twist

Persian Kabobs (page 209)

*Grilled Vegetable Tower with Feta Cheese
and Balsamic Vinegar Reduction (page 168)*

Berry Confetti Cobbler (page 239)

While we were in France, Bruce and Caroline stayed at our beach house with their friends Sydelle and Siavash, who have a little girl just about Camelia's age and a baby just about Violet's age. While we stayed in a castle, they spent the days *making* sand castles. On the Fourth of July they wanted to have a fabulous but easy lunch that was more exciting than hamburgers, hot dogs, and watermelon. Sydelle suggested they make Persian kabobs instead, which is the only way Siavash's family eats hamburgers. Persian kabobs don't come on a stick; they're just the tastiest little hamburger patties you've ever had. After you try them, you'll never make a regular hamburger again.

You start with ground beef, then shred an onion with a grater. Add the special Persian seasoning called Koubideh, and let the meat sit for eight to twenty-four hours. To make the grilled vegetables, slice eggplant, yellow peppers, onions, and tomatoes and toss them on the grill with a little olive oil.

After they're grilled, stack them in a pile and crumble feta cheese over the top. Then pour a reduction of balsamic vinegar over the top and serve with the grilled kabobs. The only thing American about this meal is the barbecue!

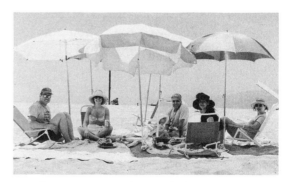

*Caroline and Bruce's 4th of July
party at our beachhouse.*

Seafood Kitchen Dinner at the Counter

Spicy Rock Shrimp Salad (page 182)

Crispy Mesquite Salmon (page 184)

Summer Stir-Fry (page 167)

As it happened, 1998 was an incredibly busy year for me: work, work, work. By the time August rolled around, I felt as though Alan and I had been running on a treadmill, and the treadmill was winning. It was time to get some balance back in my life, so we agreed to slow down and take some time for ourselves to relax. We thought about planning a vacation, but we'd just been to France and the idea of getting on yet another plane was abhorrent to both of us. Instead we decided to treat ourselves to a vacation at our lovely beach house in Los Angeles. Why not? The weather was beautiful, the accommodations were exactly to our liking, and the food was amazing . . . because we cooked it ourselves!

One evening Alan and I decided to have a lovely seafood fest at the kitchen counter. I made a delicious, spicy rock shrimp salad. Rock shrimp has a wonderful lobster flavor and combines well with the serrano chilies, cilantro, red onions, and lime juice, with the added crunch of pickling cucumbers. Exotic, spicy, and refreshing for a summer salad!

For our entrée Alan had two beautiful pieces of fresh salmon, which we encrusted with green and black peppercorns, coriander, and dill. Then Alan grilled it over a very hot mesquite fire, which adds a terrific smoky flavor. Meanwhile I made a stir-fry of summer vegetables with julienned summer squash, zucchini, bamboo shoots, and leeks. When the salmon was cooked it had this fabulous crispy crust on the top, and it tasted great served over the vegetables. A perfect summer meal at the kitchen counter with my husband. Some old adages remain constant; there is nothing like a home-cooked meal, and there is no place like home.

Sunday Night Dinner in the Dining Room

Steamed Artichokes with Lemon-Dill Dip
(EGLW, page 85)

Buffalo Mozzarella, Fennel, and Celery Salad (page 137)

Parsnip Garlic Ravioli with Mushroom Ragout (page 230)

Mountain of Lemon Meringue Pie (page 244)

Daisy and Camelia were running in circles around the kitchen. Bruce was prepping the artichokes. Leslie was setting up the art table for the girls to make collages. Caroline was nursing Violet. Alan was chopping vegetables for the salad. Frank was pulling the umbrellas off the beach as the sun slipped behind the mountain. And me? I was making homemade ravioli. It was another Sunday night dinner at the Hamel home.

I have always loved ravioli and I have found an incredible way to make it with whole-wheat wonton wrappers. They are thin and precut into squares, which makes the preparation go that much faster. Because, let's face it, ravioli is a labor of love, so spend your time making it for those who will appreciate it most.

We started the meal with steamed artichokes dipped in my signature lemon-dill mayonnaise. My family never tires of arti-

chokes! They are Bruce's favorite food. For the salad we had chopped fennel, buffalo mozzarella, and celery tossed in a light lemon-and-olive-oil dressing. For dinner I served the light and delicious parsnip ravioli with a sauce made from tomatoes and mushrooms. A stunning entrée! And to top off this Level Two meal, Mountain of Lemon Meringue Pie with the perfect combination of tart and sweet lemon curd.

As I looked around the table, I felt proud of my family. I feel fortunate to have each and every one of them in my life. Every day I learn something I didn't know the day before, and every day I have the opportunity to grow spiritually and emotionally. We just have to take the time to listen to the lessons life has to offer and to treasure the moments with our loved ones. It's exactly what Sunday dinners are made of.

My Birthday Lunch in the Somers' Garden

Jicama and Snap Pea Citrus Salad (page 137)

Chicken Breasts Stuffed with Goat Cheese–Cilantro Pesto (page 191)

Tomatillo Salsa (page 154)

Pico de Gallo (page 154)

Decadent White Chocolate Cake (page 249)

Bruce and Caroline recently completed the last step on the remodeling of their home—the landscaping. For years Bruce has been promising Caroline an English rose garden. "I beg your pardon," she would say to him, "but didn't you promise me a rose garden?" Finally their garden dream has become a reality, and their English garden couldn't be more spectacular. They put in a darling white picket fence surrounded by flowers, herbs, and vines, including fifty rosebushes of lavender, white, peach, and pink.

For my birthday in October they invited us over for lunch under the pergola in the garden. It was a magical day. We sipped beautiful frosty drinks made from pineapple and ginger as we toured the garden. The bees were pollinating the foxgloves and delphiniums. The purple trumpet vine wrapped around the posts of the pergola, winding its way to the top. The soft blue hydrangeas bloomed under the pussy willow tree. The wisteria climbed along the eaves of the backyard. Monarch butterflies danced on the flowering butterfly bushes. The tiny white roses wound through the white pickets of the fence, and the rosebushes had touches of blooms here and there, previewing the magic of their full bloom in the coming spring. A truly enchanted garden.

Lunch was equally divine. An hour after our fruit drink we had a jicama and sugar snap pea salad: crispy, light, and refreshing with red onions and a squeeze of fresh lime and lemon juice (right off the lemon tree).

The entrée consisted of chicken breasts, grilled with the skin left on, then stuffed with a mixture of goat cheese, cilantro, and serrano chilies. The combination of the creamy goat cheese and the spicy cilantro pesto makes for an incredible flavor. And the presentation was beautiful, served with Green Tomatillo Salsa and Pico de Gallo. Our mouths exploded with flavor!

And to top it off? Well, anyone who knows me knows that birthday cake is my weakness. And no better time than your own birthday to have a big "blow it" like Decadent White Chocolate Cake. Camelia and Caroline made the cake and decorated it with candied violets and tiny Australian violets picked from the garden. And my gift, on top of the amazing meal, was a set of tiny silver salt and pepper shakers for my collection. I want to get enough so that each person will have his or her own individual set. Who says you can't look forward to birthdays at my age!

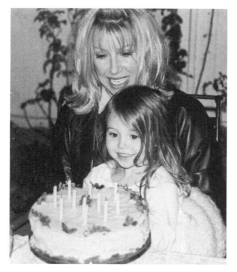

My granddaughter Camelia helped make my delicious Decadent White Chocolate Cake.

Every Thanksgiving Alan and I host a full week of food and fun for our family at our desert home. Of all the holidays, Thanksgiving is celebrated with the most fanfare. We eat incredible food all week long. We laugh and talk and swim and hike and dance and eat and eat and eat. I shared all my Thanksgiving recipes in the first book, *Eat Great, Lose Weight,* and those traditional dishes have not changed. My turkey with mushroom sausage stuffing still pleases the crowd like no other. And my pureed celery root is no longer just a substitute for mashed potatoes, it's considered a delicacy.

After everyone has cleared out from the festivities of Thanksgiving week, Alan and I take some time to ourselves to soak in all that the desert has to offer. Sometimes we sit for long periods of time without talking, just listening to the sounds of the birds and the gentle breeze blowing through the Paloverde trees. One night after just such a day, I looked in the refrigerator and thought about what I might prepare for dinner. I saw a beautiful ball of buffalo mozzarella and decided to start by slicing

that with vine-ripened tomatoes and basil. Hmmm, then dinner . . . what to make for dinner. I started by chopping an onion and browning it in olive oil. Then I added a few cloves of garlic. I had some ground turkey meat, which I added and browned. At this point I still did not know what I was making . . . but I pressed on. I went outside and clipped some thyme from the garden, then washed and chopped the leaves and added them to the ground turkey. And mushrooms . . . I use them in many meals, and I always enjoy the flavor they bring. I had shiitake mushrooms, but any variety would do. I chopped off the stems and browned them until they were crusty, then added sea salt and freshly ground pepper. Then on high heat I poured a cup of white wine and cooked it down until the steam subsided and the taste of the alcohol had dissipated. To this I added a little homemade turkey broth that I had left over from my Thanksgiving turkey. I scraped the brown bits off the bottom of the pan and let the broth cook down. I took a taste from the large wooden spoon . . . yum!

Now, what to do with it. I could serve it in a lettuce cup like a taco. The crunchiness of the lettuce would be great. Or I could carve out a zucchini, a tomato, and an onion and stuff it inside, then bake for forty minutes or so. Or I could add beaten eggs and make a scramble. Or I could pour the egg and meat into muffin tins and bake for little individual quiches. Or I could add the rest of that incredible turkey broth and have a wonderful soup. And the winner is . . . the soup! But for the next couple of days we had the scramble for breakfast, the tacos for lunch, and the baked vegetables for dinner. What a great way to use your leftovers for fast, easy meals.

I find myself making these kinds of meals frequently throughout the week. I call them "sautés." The great thing about "sautés" is that they can be made from whatever you have in your refrigerator. I always start with an onion and brown it in olive oil. Then I add whatever kind of meat, poultry, or seafood I have on hand. I season it with fresh or dried herbs, then add whatever chopped vegetables I have on hand. Then I deglaze the pan with broth or wine (or both) and scrape up those bits on the bottom of the pan. Remember, the bits are the key to flavor! Then reduce the liquid, turn off the heat, and stir in a pat of butter. It's always a winner.

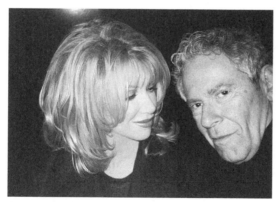

Alan is my best friend.

DECEMBER

Cooking the Christmas Goose

*Baby Greens with Pomegranates and Champagne
Vinaigrette (page 148)*

Pumpkin Soup with Roasted Shallots and Sage (page 228)

Roast Christmas Goose with Port Glaze (page 201)

Wild Rice

French-Style Green Beans

Chocolate Pots de Crème (page 238)

Christmas is one of those seasons that brings out the best of times and the worst of times. We all try to plan the perfect day . . . Christmas carols playing in the background and a beautifully set table with antique linens, china, crystal, and all the freshly polished silver. Beautifully wrapped gifts under the tree filled with exactly what each family member requested. And the best dinner you've ever made, each course more superb than the last.

But let's face it: it's tough to pull off. The season gets crazy as we try to get cards signed and mailed on time. We're frazzled with last-minute shopping, looking for something, anything, that seems an appropriate gift so we can check it off our list. We stay up practically all night on Christmas Eve doing last-minute wrapping, only to realize at two-thirty A.M. that we're out of tape. When Christmas morning arrives, the presents are opened in three minutes flat and we spend the remainder of the day rushing to get ready to drive to a family member's home, where we'll no doubt have a little Christmas tiff over who makes the best eggnog. Christmas creates stress! Our expectations are so high to create the perfect day that we are usually let down. The only thing we know for sure is that we always eat more than we should, we drink more than we should, and we spend more than we should.

So how can we avoid being frazzled and truly enjoy the season? Remember, you are only human, and you cannot do it all.

When you're invited to a friend's or family member's home and you know it's going to be difficult to split up your day to make an appearance at each location, lovingly decline. You will be surprised at how understanding people can be if you are honest. There is nothing worse than cutting your Christmas morning short, rushing to get dressed and out of the house, yet still arriving late and having to leave early to get back and prepare your own dinner. You cannot be all things to all people. Maybe this year you spend Christmas with one side of the family and the next year you spend it with the other side of the family. Try to simplify your day so that after all the preparation, you get to enjoy it, too!

Christmas at our home varies from year to year. Leslie and Frank usually spend the holiday with us as well as our dear friends Andrea and Nelson. Stephen and Olivia find it hard to travel from Paris at Christmas, and Bruce and Caroline generally spend the holiday with Caroline's family. With such a small group, I have the opportunity to make something really special. This year it was my all-time favorite Christmas dinner, roasted goose. The flavor of freshly roasted goose is uncommonly delicious. I started with a beautiful baby lettuce salad tossed with olive oil, Champagne vinegar, and fresh pomegranate seeds. Then we had delicious pumpkin soup. To accompany the goose I made wild rice, and French-style string beans tossed in butter. And for dessert Chocolate Pots de Crème, incredible chocolate pudding served in tiny porcelain pots with freshly whipped cream.

We all indulged a little on Christmas; it's a tough time of year to live on Level One. But I try not to take a chocolate out of the box every time it's passed around, and I don't sample each and every Christmas cookie. Because even though it's Christmas, we don't have to eat too much or drink too much or spend too much. Just remember this year in the middle of all the hustle and bustle to take the time to count your blessings. Our lives are filled with them. And for those things we still wish for . . . look forward to the following year and all the opportunities it will bring. Happy holidays.

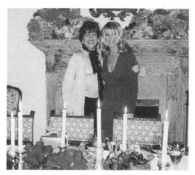

My friend Andrea and I surveying the holiday table.

Part Three

THE

SOMERSIZE

RECIPES

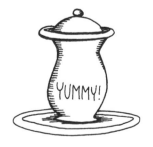

THIRTEEN

Level One Recipes

My book *Eat Great, Lose Weight* was filled with over a hundred incredible recipes. I've received letters from around the country from people who are losing weight and eating better than they've ever eaten before. The enthusiasm has been overwhelming. Many letters have requested even more Somersize recipes, and I am happy to share more than 130 new recipes with you in this book. The following Level One recipes in this chapter, as well as the Level Two recipes in the next chapter, have been developed over the last two years with great flavor in mind. You'll love making these delicious meals for your entire family. In time you will be creating your own, all the while marveling at your newly shaped body and wondering how you could possibly have ever eaten any other way. The pounds will fall off, and you'll never feel deprived or hungry.

Good luck as you *Get Skinny on Fabulous Food!*

Breakfast and Brunch

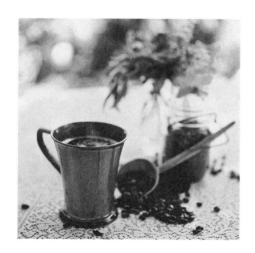

Fresh Melon Smoothie

SERVES 2

Alan, the fruitaholic, created this delicious blend. The key is finding sweet melon. There's nothing more disappointing than cutting open a melon and finding it's flavorless. Alan always asks the produce person in the market to cut the melon open so he can taste it before he buys it.

1 cup seeded ripe watermelon chunks
1 cup honeydew melon chunks
½ cup white grape juice

Juice of 1 lime
5 to 6 ice cubes

   Place the melon chunks, grape juice, and lime juice in a blender and puree until smooth. Add the ice cubes and blend until smooth and frothy. Serve immediately.

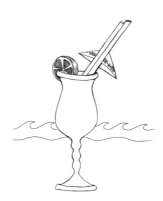

Fresh Tomato Juice

VEGGIES: LEVEL ONE

SERVES 2

Homemade tomato juice is like nectar from the gods. Make sure you have beautiful vine-ripened tomatoes.

5 medium very ripe tomatoes, halved
Salt and freshly ground black pepper

Juice of 1 lemon

Place the halved tomatoes, skin side down, in a large nonstick skillet. Drizzle with a tablespoon of water. Cover and cook over medium heat for 30 minutes. Check occasionally to make sure there is liquid in the pan. If there isn't liquid in the pan, add a little water ¼ cup at a time.

Pour the tomatoes and juice into a sieve placed over a large bowl. Mash the tomatoes with a wooden spoon to get all the pulp through the sieve without seeds and skin.

Add salt and pepper to taste and a little lemon juice. Chill and serve over ice.

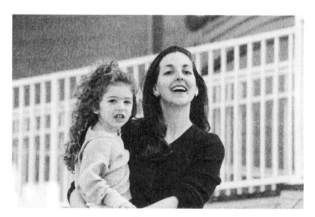

Daisy with Caroline at Camelia's birthday party.

Leslie's Mushroom, Broccoli, and Egg Cupcakes

PROTEINS/FATS AND VEGGIES: LEVEL ONE

MAKES ABOUT 10 CUPCAKES

There are so many wonderful ways to eat eggs when you Somersize. My stepdaughter, Leslie, makes delicious egg cupcakes by using omelet batter poured into cupcake tins. Her husband, Frank, eats more eggs than anyone I know. That's why we call him "Oeuf Boy." These are great to keep in the refrigerator for afternoon snacks or a fast meal. Leslie flavors them with every vegetable or meat you could imagine. Here's one of my favorites.

3 tablespoons butter
1 pound mushrooms, thinly sliced
2 cups broccoli florets
2 tablespoons olive oil

6 ounces Swiss cheese, grated
Salt and freshly ground black pepper
9 large eggs

Preheat the oven to 350°F. Grease the cupcake tins with a little olive oil.

Place a large skillet over medium-high heat. Melt the butter. Add the mushrooms and sauté until they become browned and crusty on the edges, 10 to 15 minutes. Transfer the cooked mushrooms to a food processor and blend until minced. (If you don't have a food processor, you can chop the mushrooms.)

Place the broccoli florets in a steamer basket over boiling water and steam until tender, 5 to 7 minutes. Remove the broccoli from the heat and place in a mixing bowl. Add the olive oil and mash the broc-

coli lightly with a fork until chunky. Add the sliced and minced mushrooms and the grated cheese. Season with salt and pepper. Mix well with your hands.

Fill each cupcake tin half full with the mushroom-broccoli mixture.

In a bowl, beat the eggs with a splash of water until light and fluffy. Season with salt and pepper. Pour the batter into the greased cupcake tins over the vegetables until about three quarters full.

Bake the cupcakes for approximately 10 minutes. Serve immediately or wrap each cupcake in plastic wrap and store in the refrigerator or freezer.

Breakfast Bruschetta

CARBOS AND VEGGIES: LEVEL ONE

SERVES 2

I first tasted this breakfast in Tuscany. It's fast, easy, and delicious. The key is finding great tomatoes. If your market only carries tasteless pink tomatoes, try to find a farmer's market that sells vine-ripened tomatoes. And remember, don't put tomatoes in the refrigerator or they'll get mushy.

4 slices of multigrain bread
2 ripe tomatoes, sliced
Salt and freshly ground black pepper

4 fresh basil leaves
1 sweet onion (Vidalia or Maui), thinly
    sliced (optional)

Toast or grill the bread until lightly browned. Top with beautiful ripe tomato slices, salt and pepper to taste, and fresh basil leaves. You can also use thinly sliced Vidalia onion rings on top of the tomatoes if the taste is not too strong for your palette in the morning.

For Level Two
Brush the grilled bread with a good-quality extra-virgin olive oil. It's only a minor imbalance and simply delicious.

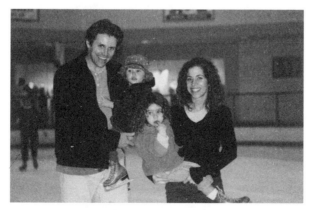

Bruce, Cornelia, Daisy, and Leslie.
Our kids are all such good friends.

Artichoke Frittata

SERVES 2

This is a great breakfast. Or try it for lunch or dinner with a simple green salad.

4 large eggs
Salt and freshly ground black pepper
2 tablespoons olive oil
2 medium onions, chopped

¾ cup marinated artichoke hearts, drained
   and chopped
Sprinkle of grated Parmesan cheese

Preheat the oven to 350°F.

Whisk the eggs in a bowl with a splash of water. Season with salt and pepper. Place a medium sauté pan (with an ovenproof handle) over medium heat. When the pan is hot, add the olive oil. Sauté the onions until browned and almost crispy, 10 to 12 minutes, then set aside half the cooked onion for a garnish. Add the drained artichoke hearts and sauté for 1 minute longer.

Add the beaten eggs to the sauté pan. Immediately sprinkle with the grated cheese and remove from the heat.

Place the pan in the preheated oven. (If you do not have a sauté pan with an ovenproof handle, transfer the egg mixture at this point to a small casserole dish or pie pan.) Bake for 7 to 10 minutes, until puffy and golden. Garnish with the reserved crispy onions and serve.

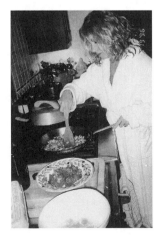

Nothing better than Artichoke Frittata after my morning swim.

Deviled Eggs

PROTEINS/FATS AND VEGGIES: LEVEL ONE

MAKES 12

Pure comfort food . . . and great for an afternoon snack.

6 large eggs
1 to 2 tablespoons mayonnaise
¼ teaspoon dry mustard (optional)

Salt and freshly ground black pepper
1 bunch of chives, finely chopped
Paprika

To hard-boil the eggs, put them in a saucepan and cover with cold water. Place over medium-high heat and bring to a boil. Reduce the heat a little until the water reaches a low boil and cook for 15 minutes.

Drain and run the eggs under cold water. Set aside to let the eggs cool.

When cooled, peel the shells from the eggs. Slice the eggs in half, lengthwise. Place all the yolks in a small mixing bowl. Add the mayonnaise, dry mustard, if desired, and salt and pepper to taste. Mash together with a fork until smooth and well combined.

Arrange the egg whites on a platter with the cavity side up. Spoon some of the filling into each hole until all are filled. Top with chopped chives and a sprinkle of paprika. Refrigerate until ready to serve.

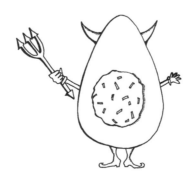

Huevos Rancheros

PROTEINS/FATS AND VEGGIES: LEVEL ONE

SERVES 2

Here's a great way to start your day.

1 tablespoon olive oil
2 onions, thinly sliced
1 5-ounce can Ortega sliced chilies
1 tomato, seeded and diced
2 tablespoons (¼ stick) butter

4 large eggs
2 ounces sharp Cheddar cheese, grated
Salsa
¼ cup sour cream
2 green onions, chopped

Heat a skillet over high heat. Add the olive oil and onions. Sauté the onions until brown and crispy, about 15 minutes. Drain the chilies and add to the onions. Add the tomato and stir until heated through. Divide onto 2 plates.

Add the butter and melt. Crack the eggs and fry them in the butter. Cover with a lid for 2 minutes to cook the whites. If you prefer the yolks cooked, keep on the heat a little longer. Repeat with the other two eggs.

Place 2 fried eggs on each plate over the onions. Top with the grated Cheddar cheese, salsa, sour cream, and green onions.

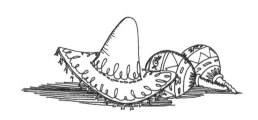

Alan's Fried Eggs in Onion Nests

PROTEINS/FATS AND VEGGIES: LEVEL ONE

SERVES 2

If you find yourself occasionally craving the taste of hash browns or home fries, this is the perfect breakfast to have. It's a Level One breakfast, but you'll think you're cheating. It's great with Alan's Awesome Bacon (page 116).

2 large onions
4 tablespoons olive oil

Salt and freshly ground black pepper
4 large eggs

To make the onion nests, peel the skin off the onions and slice as thinly as possible with a sharp knife, or use a mandoline to get very thin slices. In a large skillet, heat 1 tablespoon of olive oil over medium–high heat. When the oil is hot, add the sliced onions. Let them cook until they are brown and crispy, almost burned. (Depending on your stove, this could take 10 to 15 minutes or more.) Season with salt and pepper. Scrape the onions up with a spatula and place 2 piles on each plate. Create the "nests" by using a fork to push out the center of each pile of onions and build up the sides.

To fry the eggs, add the remaining 3 tablespoons of olive oil to the same skillet used to cook the onions and heat over medium–high heat. To test when the oil is hot enough for the eggs, add a drop of water. If it spatters and evaporates immediately, the skillet is hot enough. Crack 2 eggs, one at a time, and drop them into the hot skillet. Let the eggs cook until the whites start to brown on the edges. Then cover the skillet with a lid and cook for 1 minute longer. When you lift the lid, the whites will be cooked all the way through and the yolks will be runny. (If you prefer the yolks cooked more, leave the lid on until the yolks are cooked to your liking.) Lift the eggs out with a spatula and place 1 egg on each onion nest. Repeat the process with the last 2 eggs.

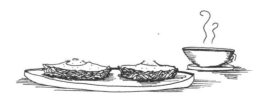

Alan's Awesome Bacon

PROTEINS/FATS: LEVEL ONE

SERVES 5

Bacon is one of those foods that has been taboo in our fat-free society. No longer! When you Somersize you can freely enjoy the incredible flavor of bacon . . . and no one makes it more incredible than Alan. We like to sprinkle this bacon all around our egg dishes. And it's a perfect garnish for Alan's Fried Eggs in Onion Nests (page 115). Make sure to look for nitrate-free bacon for a healthier option.

1 pound bacon

2 tablespoons olive oil

Cut the bacon strips into ½-inch pieces. Heat a large skillet over medium-high heat. Add the olive oil and heat for a minute or two. Add the bacon and fry until golden brown, gently separating the pieces by stirring with a wooden spoon. Remove the bacon from the skillet and place it on paper towels to absorb the grease.

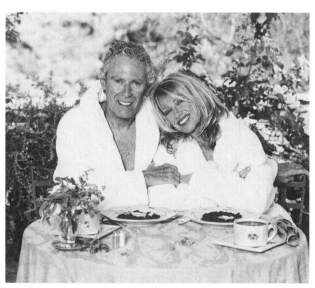

Alan's awesome bacon is perfect with scrumptious eggs in onion nests.

Perfect Cup of Decaf
LEVEL ONE

With caffeine consciousness at an all-time high, the need to learn to make and enjoy good decaf has finally arrived. One of the most significant factors in brewing coffee of any kind is the freshness of the bean and the taste of the water.

I have a palette that loves a robust, flavorful coffee. Starbucks Decaf Colombian and Guatemalan are two of my favorites and are easy to find. If you don't have a Starbucks near you, try their mail-order service. I buy whole beans and grind them myself; however, preground beans are fine as long as they are in a vacuum-sealed package. Air is the worst violator of coffee. I always refrigerate the beans and keep them in an airtight container.

Everyone has a different opinion on how to brew coffee. My favorite way is to use a drip cone over a glass pot with a brown natural coffee filter. If possible, always use purified water.

Place the coffee grounds into the filter. Alan and I like strong coffee—1 heaping tablespoon of drip grind coffee per every 8-ounce coffee cup you are going to fill. Bring the water to a boil and then turn off the burner. When the water stops bubbling and becomes still, start pouring into the coffee grounds.

When pouring hot water into a coffee filter, be very careful never to let the hot water stop until you have made all you want. That way, the grounds never settle to the bottom of the filter. You can get good results with other coffee devices as well. Tap water and old, cheap coffee beans will not make good coffee. I find that when I add hot water, a foam starts on top of the coffee. That means the beans are really fresh and there's still oxygen in them. When I find beans like that, I cherish them. Great beans made in this process make the greatest decaf money can buy. Your body will never know it is going without caffeine.

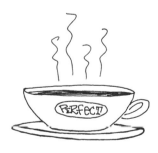

Soups and Sandwiches

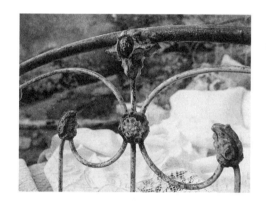

Quick Stocks

One of the most exciting parts of Somersizing is enjoying great sauces. The wine reductions and sauces in this book will wow even the toughest critic; however, there is one crucial element when it comes to sauces: stock. In order to make an incredible soup or sauce, you must start with incredible stock. That's why, whenever possible, I always make my stocks from scratch. Follow some of the recipes in my book or one of your own. And make plenty. Basic stock can take hours to prepare, so here are some tips on how to create perfect ones.

1. Think about bones. Bones store flavor. For a flavorful stock you need lots of bones. If I'm going to roast chicken, I prefer to use a whole chicken. Not only is it more economical, it tastes better and you have the added benefit of a leftover carcass to make stock. I usually roast the chicken, serve the legs and breast meat for dinner, then use the remaining meat and bones to make stock. Often the butcher will give me extra necks and backs, at no additional charge, to add to my stock. Or, for example, if I prepare a pork roast, I always cook it with the bone for extra flavor. To make serving easier, I have my butcher cut the bone off the roast, then tie it back around the meat. The roasted bones make the pan drippings fabulous and they make the most incredible stock. For fish stock I use a whole fish or just the heads and tails. It's important to check for freshness. Look at the fish's eyes. If they are cloudy, the fish is old. No matter what you make, it will not taste good.

2. Besides the bones, plenty of vegetables and herbs make stock taste great. I have given specific vegetables with amounts in the following recipes, but my own stocks will vary greatly. That's because every time I make stock I use it as an opportunity to clean out my refrigerator. If the celery has gotten a little rubbery, it's no longer good for salads, but it's perfect for stock. Older onions get tossed in. They give the stock a rich, dark color. Leeks add great flavor. The tough ends of asparagus that most cut off and throw away are great in stock. And don't forget bundles and bundles of herbs. With chicken, I love lots of thyme and parsley. If I can't spare an entire bunch of herbs for stock, I will cut off the stems to use in the stock and reserve the fresh leaves for cooking. With stock there's no need to trim the tops and bottoms off your vegetables before they get thrown in the stockpot. Just make sure they are free of dirt and sand, then cut them in half and add them to the pot.

3. Most of my recipes for stock cook from 3 to 12 hours. I prefer to cook closer to 12 hours, simmering uncovered until the liquid is reduced by one third to one half. This makes double-strength stock. After

straining the stock through a sieve, I store it in dated plastic containers in the freezer.

4. When I don't have time to make stock from scratch, I use canned broth. Make sure to check for hidden sugars and starches in canned broth. I like Hain Brand because it's all natural and tastes good in a pinch. To make it taste even better, refortify it. For instance, if I want chicken stock, I buy a large can of chicken broth, add a 5-pound whole roasting chicken to it, and cook for about a half hour. It adds tons of flavor to the canned broth. Then I remove the chicken and use the shredded chicken meat for salads or soups.

5. Another way to make good stocks is to invest in a pressure cooker or slow cooker. A pressure cooker helps infuse the flavors. An average stock takes a minimum of 3 hours, but with a pressure cooker, it takes about 30 minutes once it comes to pressure. With a slow cooker you can throw in all the ingredients in the morning when you leave for work. When you come home, you will have a splendid stock.

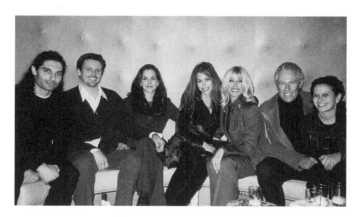

On the town in L.A.—Frank, Bruce, Caroline, Leslie, me, Alan, and our friend Amanda at Leslie's birthday dinner.

Fish Stock

MAKES ABOUT 6 CUPS

Fish stock is very important in making wonderful sauces and soups. The two key things to making excellent fish stock are: (1) procure very fresh fish and (2) do not boil the fish parts; slowly simmer the carcass.

The best way to ensure really fresh fish is to check the eyes. If the fish has a film over the eyes, it's been around awhile. The fish must have clear eyes, or it's going to smell and not taste good. I use a mild white fish because I only want a subtle taste of fish. My preference is snapper or grouper, but cod or orange roughy is good. Never use an oily-type fish such as mackerel.

2 fresh fish heads and tails (sometimes your fishmonger will give them to you)
1 cup dry white wine
1 leek, cut in half lengthwise

2 celery stalks
1 tablespoon salt
1 tablespoon paprika

Place all the ingredients, which should be cold, with 8 cups of water into a stockpot over medium-low heat. Again, never boil. Let simmer 2 to 3 hours. Drain the stock through a fine sieve, then discard the fish and vegetables. Place in plastic containers and store in the refrigerator or freezer.

Rich Capon Stock

MAKES ABOUT 3 CUPS

Capon neck and giblets
2 chicken legs
2 to 3 celery stalks

1 whole onion
1 leek, halved lengthwise and washed
Salt and freshly ground black pepper

In a medium stockpot, place the neck and giblets from inside the cavity of the capon. Then add 2 chicken legs. Cover with about 4 cups of water. Add the celery, onion, leek, and salt and pepper.

Bring to a boil. Then reduce the heat to low and continue to cook for 1 hour. After 1 hour, turn the heat up to high and reduce for 20 minutes to pull all the flavor out of the meat and vegetables. Turn off the heat and strain.

Quick Rich Chicken Stock

PROTEINS/FATS AND VEGGIES: LEVEL ONE

MAKES ABOUT 8 CUPS

If you don't have hours to spare to make a deep rich chicken stock, try this recipe. The addition of veal and beef bones give this chicken stock a rich flavor in a short amount of time.

1 5- to 6-pound whole chicken (organic, hormone-free, if possible)
1 veal bone
1 beef bone
1 piece of pancetta
1 bunch of celery, cut into pieces
1 red onion
2 tomatoes
1 head of garlic
6 bay leaves
6 fresh thyme sprigs
1 teaspoon black peppercorns
Salt

Remove any fatty parts of the chicken. Rinse the bird and place in a large stockpot with all the other ingredients, except salt, and 8 cups of water. Bring to a gentle boil over medium-high heat. Turn down the heat and skim any foam from the top. Simmer for about 1 hour. Strain the stock through a fine sieve. Remove the chicken and set aside for another meal. Discard the meat and vegetables. Season with salt. Store the stock in plastic containers in the refrigerator or freezer.

When the stock is thoroughly chilled, fat will rise to the top and harden. Remove all the fat with a spatula.

For Level Two
Add a parsnip or carrot for extra flavor.

Beef Stock

MAKES ABOUT 10 CUPS

I never like to be without this in my freezer. Your sauces and soups are only as good as your stock.

2 beef shanks
4 large short ribs
1 cup dry red wine
4 celery stalks, with tops
1 medium onion

4 garlic cloves
10 black peppercorns
1 tablespoon salt
2 thyme sprigs
1 rosemary sprig

Preheat the oven to 350°F.

Place the beef shanks and short ribs in a roasting pan and roast for 30 minutes. Remove the shanks and ribs and place in a large stockpot. Place the roasting pan on the stove over medium-high heat. When the pan is hot, add the wine and continue stirring, scraping the bits off the bottom of the pan to release the flavor. Pour the contents of the roasting pan into the stockpot.

Add all the other ingredients and 6 cups of water and cook over medium-low heat.

The stock should cook for 3 to 12 hours. The longer you cook it, the richer the stock.

Strain the stock through a fine sieve. Discard the meat and vegetables. Store the stock in plastic containers in the refrigerator or freezer.

When the stock is thoroughly chilled, fat will rise to the top and harden. Remove all the fat with a spatula.

For Level Two
Add a parsnip or carrot for extra flavor.

Roasted Chicken Stock

MAKES ABOUT 10 CUPS

They say the best cooks always have homemade stock in the freezer. Stock is the base for wonderful soups and sauces. This recipe is particularly rich and delicious because it starts with a whole roasted chicken. I use the chicken meat to make Tarragon Chicken Salad in Lettuce Cups (EGLW, page 118) or Chicken Tomato Cilantro Soup (EGLW, page 126).

1 6-pound roasting chicken (organic, hormone-free, if possible)
4 celery stalks, with tops
1 large onion
4 thyme sprigs

1 tablespoon fresh rosemary
Salt and freshly ground black pepper
1 cup dry white wine
1 bunch of parsley
1 tablespoon kosher salt

Preheat the oven to 500°F.

Remove the giblets and neck from the cavity of the chicken and put them in a roasting pan. Rinse the bird and stuff the large cavity with celery stalks and half the onion. Place the other onion half under the tail flap. Stuff the thyme and rosemary under the skin of the breast.

Sprinkle the bird with salt and pepper to taste and roast for 10 minutes. Lower the oven temperature to 325°F. and roast for 1 hour 50 minutes (20 minutes per pound). Remove the chicken and set it aside.

Pour the contents of the roasting pan (the neck, giblets, and pan drippings) into an 8-quart stockpot. Be sure to get every last bit off the bottom of the roasting pan. Add all the remaining ingredients to the stockpot with 12 cups of water and let come to a boil.

Remove the skin from the chicken and discard. Remove large pieces of meat and put away for later. Split the bones with a mallet and add to the stock. Bring the stock back to a boil, being careful to skim off any foam that comes to the top.

The stock should simmer for at least 3 hours, preferably 12 hours, to get a deep, dark stock. Strain the stock through a fine sieve. Discard the bones and vegetables. Store the stock in plastic containers in the refrigerator or freezer. Remove the fat after it solidifies.

For Level Two
Add a parsnip or carrot for extra flavor.

Roasted Vegetable Stock

VEGGIES: LEVEL ONE

MAKES ABOUT 6 CUPS

This is a great stock to use for Level One Carbo recipes because it's made without any protein or fat. Of course it can be used for Pro/Fats recipes as well because it's made from all vegetables. The stock gets extra flavor from roasting the vegetables.

1 red bell pepper
4 celery stalks, with tops
1 medium sweet onion
2 small turnips
1 medium parsnip (see Note)
1 small rutabaga
1 tablespoon kosher salt

3 garlic cloves
1 leek
1 cup dry white wine
1 bunch of parsley
8 thyme sprigs
10 black peppercorns
1 teaspoon paprika

Preheat the oven to 350°F.

Place the pepper, celery, onion, turnips, parsnip, and rutabaga in a baking dish. Sprinkle with salt. Place the dish in the oven and roast the vegetables for 30 minutes.

Place the roasted vegetables, 8 cups of water, and all the remaining ingredients into a stockpot. Make sure you scrape all the bits from the baking dish. Simmer for 1½ hours.

Strain the stock through a fine sieve, making sure you squeeze the juice out of the vegetables. Discard the vegetables.

Note

Parsnips are technically a Funky Food, but using just one in this stock will create an imbalance so minor, I would not worry about it.

Greek Lemon Pepper Chicken Soup

PROTEINS/FATS AND VEGGIES: LEVEL ONE

SERVES 6

This soup is great when made from the leftover carcass from my Crunchy Roasted Lemon Chicken (page 196). For the quick version, buy 2 large cans of chicken broth and a rotisserie chicken from the deli.

STOCK

1 chicken carcass
4 celery stalks
2 garlic cloves
2 shallots
1 bunch of parsley
6 black peppercorns
2 teaspoons fresh tarragon (or 1 teaspoon dried)
1 cup dry white wine

SOUP

2 tablespoons olive oil
1 medium onion, chopped
3 large eggs, beaten
1 cup chopped fresh spinach
1 cup lemon juice
1 lemon, thinly sliced
Shaved Parmesan cheese

To make the stock, remove most of the meat from the chicken carcass. Cut the bones in half if you have a big butcher knife; otherwise, leave them whole. Put the bones in a 5-quart stockpot. If you have sauce left over from the Crunchy Roasted Lemon Chicken, add to the bones. Add the celery, garlic, shallots, parsley, peppercorns, tarragon, 6 cups of water, and the wine. Bring to a boil, then lower the heat and simmer, uncovered, for 3 to 12 hours. The longer you cook it, the richer the stock.

Strain the stock through a fine sieve. Discard the meat and vegetables. Store the stock in plastic containers in the refrigerator. When the stock is thoroughly chilled, fat will rise to the top and harden. Remove the fat and discard.

To make the soup, place a stockpot over medium-high heat. Add the olive oil and onion. Sauté the onion until transparent, about 4 minutes. Add the stock and bring to a boil. Slowly add the beaten eggs, stirring constantly. Add any leftover chicken pieces along with the spinach. When the spinach is wilted, add the lemon juice and bring to a boil. Serve in bowls with a slice of lemon floating on top and Parmesan shavings.

Broccoli Soup

SERVES 4 TO 6

Soup made from fresh vegetables is a real treat. This recipe, made from broccoli, takes only 25 minutes to prepare. It's a great way to start a meal. This can easily become an all-Veggies recipe if you substitute Roasted Vegetable Stock (page 126) for the chicken stock. In that case, you could serve it with Carbos and garnish with a little nonfat yogurt instead of sour cream.

2 tablespoons (¼ stick) butter
1 head of broccoli, chopped
4 cups chicken stock (pages 123 and 125)
Salt and freshly ground black pepper

GARNISH

6 tablespoons sour cream (optional)
1 small bunch of chives (optional)

Place a large skillet over low heat. Add the butter and stir until just melted. Add the broccoli and sauté until tender, about 7 minutes. Add the chicken stock and bring to a boil. Lower the heat and simmer for 20 minutes.

If you have a hand mixer, like the Braun hand mixer, you can put it directly in the soup pot and puree the broccoli. I like to leave the soup slightly chunky. If you do not have a hand mixer, take 2 cups of the cooked soup and put it into a food processor or blender to puree. Add the second 2 cups and partially puree so the soup will be a little chunky. Add salt and pepper to taste.

Serve immediately. Garnish with the sour cream and sprinkle with the snipped fresh chives, if desired.

Cauliflower Soup

SERVES 4 TO 6

Cauliflower is an underrated vegetable. I love its unique flavor and texture. Like Broccoli Soup (page 128), this takes only 25 minutes to prepare. This can easily become an all-Veggies recipe if you substitute Roasted Vegetable Stock (page 126) for the chicken stock. In that case, you could serve it with Carbos and garnish with a little nonfat yogurt instead of sour cream.

2 tablespoons (¼ stick) butter
1 head of cauliflower, chopped
4 cups chicken stock (pages 123 and 125)
Salt and freshly ground black pepper

GARNISH

6 tablespoons sour cream (optional)
1 small bunch of chives (optional)

Place a skillet over medium heat. Add the butter and stir until just melted. Add the cauliflower and sauté until tender, about 7 minutes. Add the chicken stock and bring to a boil. Lower the heat and simmer for 20 minutes.

If you have a hand mixer, like the Braun hand mixer, you can put it directly in the soup pot and puree the cauliflower. I like to leave the soup slightly chunky. If you do not have a hand mixer, take 2 cups of the cooked soup and put it into a food processor or blender to puree. Add the second 2 cups and partially puree so the soup will be a little chunky. Add salt and pepper to taste.

Serve immediately. Garnish with the sour cream and sprinkle with the snipped fresh chives, if desired.

Turkey and Shiitake Mushroom Soup

PROTEINS/FATS AND VEGGIES: LEVEL ONE

SERVES 8

I discovered this recipe while cleaning out my refrigerator. I just kept adding a little of this and a little of that. Now it's a regular at our house.

2 tablespoons olive oil
2 onions, chopped
1 pound shiitake mushrooms (button mushrooms can be substituted), thinly sliced
Salt and freshly ground black pepper
1 tablespoon chopped fresh tarragon
2 pounds ground dark turkey
¼ cup dry white wine

1 tablespoon butter
½ cup sliced celery
6 cups fresh or canned chicken broth (if using canned broth, try to find unsalted)
2 zucchini, chopped into bite-size pieces

GARNISH

¼ cup grated Parmesan cheese (optional)

Place a medium stockpot over high heat. Add the olive oil and onions and stir constantly until the onions start to brown. Then turn down the heat to medium and continue stirring until the onions turn a deep golden brown and begin to caramelize, about 15 minutes. When the onions are almond colored, add the mushrooms. Season with salt and pepper and the tarragon. Stir constantly until the mushrooms get brown and crusty, 7 to 10 minutes.

Add the ground turkey a little at a time, using your fingers to break it up. Add additional salt and pepper. Brown the meat for about 5 minutes, stirring constantly. Pour in the white wine. Cook until the steam subsides and the alcohol is burned off, about 5 minutes. Scrape the bits off the bottom of the pan to release the flavors. Add the butter and celery, stirring to combine. Add the chicken broth. Bring to a boil, then lower the heat and let the soup simmer for about 15 minutes. Add the chopped zucchini and simmer 5 minutes more.

Serve in soup bowls with freshly grated Parmesan cheese, if desired.

Sweet Vidalia French Onion Soup

SERVES 4

This delicious soup is made from sweet onions and beef broth for a deep dark stock. I use a portobello mushroom cap instead of a piece of bread to hold the Gruyère cheese and it's even better than the traditional way. It'll warm your tummy and your soul. It's best with homemade Beef Stock (page 124), but canned works fine in a pinch.

3 medium sweet onions (Maui or Vidalia)
2 tablespoons olive oil, plus extra for brushing
Salt and freshly ground black pepper
1 teaspoon mustard seed
1 teaspoon celery seed

1 teaspoon cracked black pepper
4 cups beef stock or consommé
1/4 cup red wine
1 tablespoon Worcestershire sauce (see Note)
1 large portobello mushroom
4 slices of Gruyère or provolone cheese

Slice the onions very thinly with a sharp knife or a mandoline. Place a 5-quart stockpot over medium-high heat. Add the olive oil and the onions. After about 10 minutes, lower the heat to medium-low. Add salt and pepper to taste, mustard seed, celery seed, and cracked pepper and continue to sauté the onions until caramelized to a deep golden brown, another 20 to 25 minutes.

When the onions are a rich brown, add the beef stock, wine, and Worcestershire sauce. Turn the heat up to medium and cook for about 15 minutes.

Preheat the broiler.

In the meantime, cut the stem off the portobello mushroom. Place the mushroom cap on its side and slice into 4 round thin pieces. Heat a large skillet over medium-high heat.

Brush the mushroom slices with olive oil and place in the skillet, cooking for a couple of minutes on each side until lightly browned.

Ladle the soup into ovenproof bowls. Place a mushroom slice on top and then a slice of Gruyère cheese. This soup is best when served in stoneware or other ovenproof soup bowls, because you can then place the bowls on a cookie sheet under the broiler for a minute or two and let the cheese get brown and bubbly.

Note
Worcestershire sauce has a little sugar in it, but we're using such a small amount that it creates only the slightest imbalance. If you are doing well on Level One, feel free to add it.

B.L.T.

SERVES 2

Whoever said a B.L.T. had to have bread? With this yummy combination, you won't miss it. I like to serve this in iceberg lettuce cups. For a more elegant presentation, try endive leaves or radicchio cups.

6 slices of bacon
1 head of iceberg lettuce

3 to 4 tablespoons mayonnaise
2 ripe medium tomatoes, chopped

To cook the bacon, place a small skillet over medium-high heat. Add the bacon and fry until golden brown. Turn off the heat, then remove the bacon and place on paper towels to absorb the grease. When cooled, crumble into small pieces.

Make 6 lettuce "cups" by carefully peeling the leaves off of the head, trying to keep them whole. Chop the remaining lettuce into thin strips.

To assemble the B.L.T., arrange 3 lettuce cups on each plate. Spread as much mayonnaise as you like onto each. Place a small handful of chopped lettuce into each cup. Add the chopped tomatoes, evenly dividing them among the lettuce cups. Top with the crumbled bacon. Fold up like a taco and enjoy.

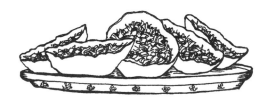

Veggie Wrap

CARBOS AND VEGGIES: LEVEL ONE

SERVES 4

Whole-wheat lavash or tortillas make great wraps filled with vegetables and nonfat cheese. You'll love this when you're craving a Carbo meal. Serve it with Cucumber Salad (page 136).

1 eggplant, sliced paper thin
2 medium zucchini, sliced paper thin
4 pieces of whole-wheat lavash bread (or 4 whole-wheat fat-free tortillas)
1 cup nonfat ricotta cheese

Salt and freshly ground black pepper
2 Roasted Red Peppers (*EGLW,* page 81), or a jar of roasted peppers in water
4 red leaf lettuce leaves

Preheat the oven to 350°F.

Salt the eggplant and the zucchini slices on both sides and place in a colander to let the excess water drain. Rinse and pat dry. Place the slices in a single layer on cookie sheets. Bake for approximately 20 minutes. Remove any smaller pieces as they become brown, so as not to burn any of the slices.

Lay the lavash or tortilla flat on a chopping block. Spread the ricotta cheese in a thin layer over the entire piece of bread. Season with salt and pepper. Place the eggplant in a single layer over the ricotta. Then place a single layer of the zucchini. Place the roasted red peppers in a single row down the middle. Top with a lettuce leaf. Roll up the bread or tortilla and secure with a toothpick (or use a tiny bit of water to "glue" the tortilla to the other side). Slice on the diagonal and serve.

Caesar Salad Sandwich

SERVES 2

Sandwiches seem perplexing while Somersizing, but remember, whole wheat bread and vegetables make incredible sandwiches. Use your imagination—thin slices of onion, peppers, crunchy lettuce, crusty bakery bread. It's hard to go wrong. This is particularly yummy. I make my Candied Tomatoes without any oil for this Level One sandwich. Just bake tomato halves at 350°F. for about 3 hours with a sprinkle of thyme.

8 Candied Tomatoes (*EGLW,* page 76)
1 head of romaine lettuce, chopped
1 red onion, thinly sliced
1 garlic clove, minced
1 tablespoon balsamic vinegar

Salt and freshly ground black pepper
1 lemon wedge
1 whole-wheat or multigrain baguette,
    lightly toasted

In a bowl, toss together the tomatoes, chopped lettuce, onion slices, garlic, balsamic vinegar, and salt and pepper. Squeeze a little lemon juice over all and toss. Taste and adjust the seasonings.

Pile onto fresh crusty multigrain bread. Put the top on the sandwich, cut in half, and eat immediately.

For Level Two
Eliminate the balsamic vinegar and toss the ingredients in Caesar Salad Dressing (*EGLW,* page 117) with grated Parmesan cheese.

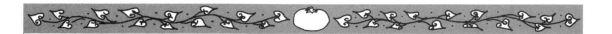

Salads

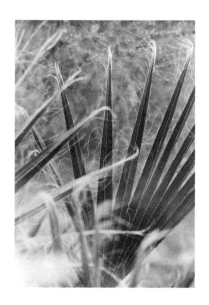

Cucumber Salad

CARBOS AND VEGGIES: LEVEL ONE

SERVES 4

My housekeeper, Shanti, makes this cool and refreshing salad. I love it alongside my Veggie Wrap (page 133). If you are eating a Carbo meal you should use this version, made the traditional way with nonfat yogurt. If you are eating a Pro/Fats meal use the version below.

2 cups nonfat yogurt
1 cucumber, peeled and thinly sliced

1 sweet onion, thinly sliced

Combine all ingredients in a bowl. Chill and serve.

Cucumber Salad

PROTEINS/FATS AND VEGGIES: LEVEL ONE

SERVES 4

Since yogurt has carbohydrates, you cannot eat it with Pro/Fats. But I love this salad with spicy meats, like Persian Kabobs (page 209) and Shanti's Chicken Curry (page 194), so I substitute crème fraîche, which has no carbohydrates, for the yogurt. Crème fraîche can be found in gourmet markets, or you can make your own using my simple recipe. It's nice and tangy like yogurt.

2 cups crème fraîche (page 152)
1 cucumber, peeled and thinly sliced

1 sweet onion, thinly sliced

Combine all ingredients in a bowl. Chill and serve.

Jicama and Snap Pea Citrus Salad
PROTEINS/FATS AND VEGGIES: LEVEL ONE

SERVES 4

This crunchy salad tastes fresh and delicious with lemon and lime juice. The red onions turn a fabulous neon color after marinating in the lime juice.

1 red onion, sliced paper thin
Juice of 6 limes
Salt

2 cups jicama, peeled and cut into julienne
2 cups sugar snap peas, cut into julienne
1 recipe Lemon-Mint Vinaigrette (page 139)

Marinate the thinly sliced red onion in the lime juice with a little salt and let stand for a few hours.

Combine the jicama and sugar snap peas.

Toss with the vinaigrette. Place on salad plates and garnish each with a handful of the marinated onions.

Buffalo Mozzarella, Fennel, and Celery Salad
PROTEINS/FATS AND VEGGIES: LEVEL ONE

SERVES 4

I tasted this at an Italian restaurant in New York and just loved the crunchiness of the celery and fennel with the smooth buffalo mozzarella. Here's my best replication.

1 fennel bulb, trimmed and chopped
4 celery stalks, chopped
1 8-ounce ball buffalo mozzarella or whole-milk mozzarella, chopped into bite-size pieces

Juice of 1 lemon
1/4 cup extra-virgin olive oil
Salt and freshly ground black pepper

Place the fennel, celery, and mozzarella in a salad bowl. Toss with the lemon juice, olive oil, and salt and pepper to taste. Serve immediately.

Lamb's Lettuce Salad with Warmed Goat Cheese

PROTEINS/FATS AND VEGGIES: LEVEL ONE

SERVES 6

Lamb's lettuce, also known as mâche, is a delicate, sweet lettuce. If you can't find it, use watercress, arugula, butter lettuce, endive, or a combination of all.

1 cup extra-virgin olive oil
2 garlic cloves, crushed
Salt and freshly ground black pepper
12 fresh basil leaves

12 1-inch-thick slices of mild goat cheese
½ cup grated Romano cheese
1 pound mâche
1 recipe Herb Vinaigrette (page 155)

In a mixing cup, combine the oil, garlic, salt and pepper to taste, and basil. Place the goat cheese in a shallow dish and pour the oil over it. Let marinate for at least 1 hour, basting frequently.

Preheat the oven to 450°F. Remove the cheese from the oil, reserving the oil for the dressing. Coat the goat cheese with the grated Romano on both sides and place on a baking sheet. Bake for 6 to 10 minutes, until the cheese begins to bubble.

Toss the mâche with the dressing and arrange on 6 plates. Place 2 slices of the warmed goat cheese on each plate and serve immediately.

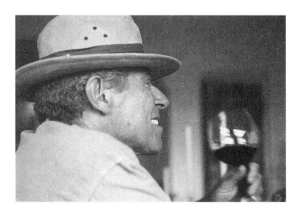

My pal Al. Such a great husband.

Garden Greens with Pear Tomatoes and Lemon-Mint Vinaigrette

PROTEINS/FATS AND VEGGIES: LEVEL ONE

SERVES 6

This light salad has the refreshing tastes of lemon and mint.

½ head of red leaf lettuce, washed and
   dried
1 head of butter lettuce, washed and dried
1 small head of frisée (curly baby endive)
1 carton yellow pear-shaped or cherry
   tomatoes

LEMON-MINT VINAIGRETTE

¼ cup white wine vinegar
1 tablespoon chopped fresh mint leaves
Salt and freshly ground black pepper
½ cup extra-virgin olive oil

GARNISH

Lemon zest

Tear the lettuces into bite-size pieces. Combine them with the tomatoes in a large salad bowl.

For the vinaigrette, whisk together the vinegar, mint leaves, and salt and pepper to taste in a mixing cup. Add the oil in a slow stream, whisking constantly until the oil is emulsified.

Toss the salad with the dressing. Garnish with the lemon zest and serve immediately.

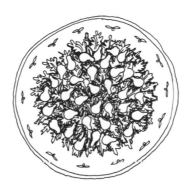

Chanterelle Salad with Creamy Parmesan Dressing (Insalata di Finferli con Crema di Parmigiano)

PROTEINS/FATS AND VEGGIES: LEVEL ONE

SERVES 4

There is a corner restaurant in Beverly Hills called Il Pastaio. The chef, Giacomino Drago, makes a special salad with chanterelle mushrooms. Here's his recipe for perfection.

½ pound arugula
3 heads of Belgian endive, chopped
1 Roma tomato, chopped
½ red onion, thinly sliced
1 tablespoon olive oil
3 ounces chanterelle mushrooms

CREAMY PARMESAN DRESSING

1 large egg
1½ tablespoons mayonnaise
1 tablespoon Dijon mustard
1 tablespoon anchovy paste
1 tablespoon minced garlic

1 tablespoon Worcestershire sauce (see Note, page 131)
1 tablespoon red wine vinegar
1 teaspoon hot pepper sauce
1½ tablespoons fresh lemon juice
Salt and freshly ground black pepper
1½ teaspoons pomace oil (or extra-virgin olive oil)
1½ tablespoons warm water
3 tablespoons grated Parmesan cheese

GARNISH

Shaved Parmesan cheese

Combine the arugula, endive, tomato, and onion in a large salad bowl.

Place a skillet over medium-high heat and add the olive oil. Sauté the chanterelle mushrooms for 5 to 7 minutes. Remove from the heat and set aside to cool.

Meanwhile, to make the dressing, bring a small saucepan of water to a boil. Add an egg and cook for 30 seconds. Remove the egg with a slotted spoon. When cool enough to touch, crack the egg and place the yolk only in a mixing bowl. Discard the remainder. Add all ingredients except the oil, water, and Parmesan. Whisk until well combined. Then add the oil and water and whisk until emulsified. Last, stir in the grated cheese.

Add the mushrooms to the salad and toss with the dressing. Garnish with shaved Parmesan cheese. Serve immediately.

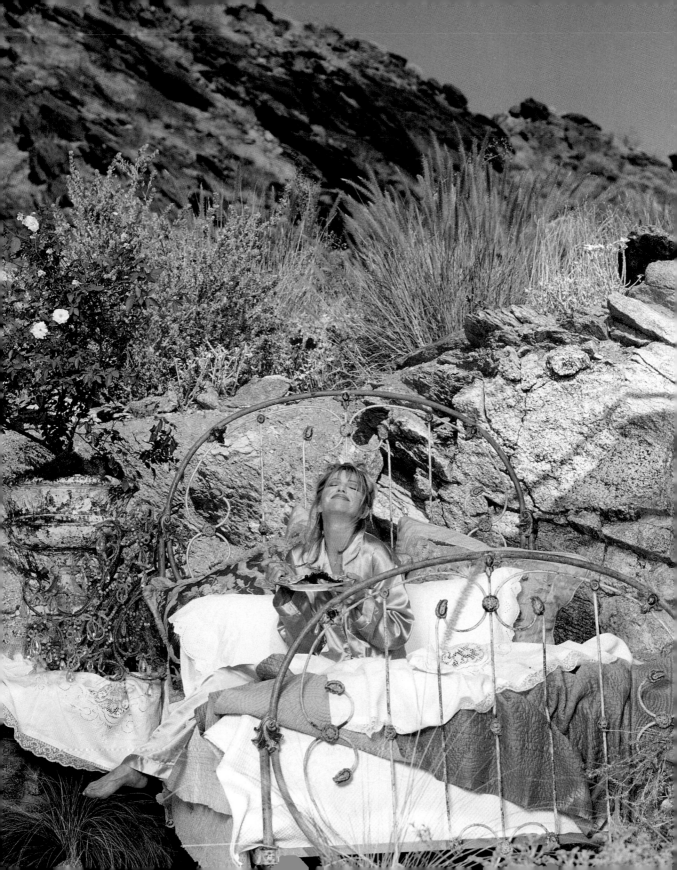

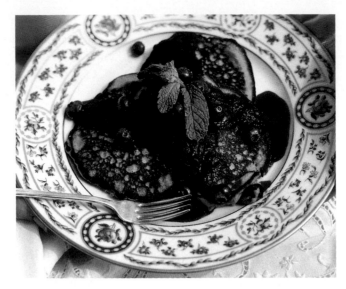

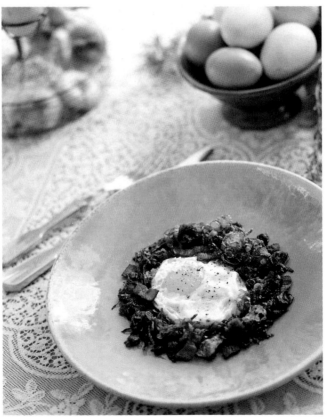

PREVIOUS PAGE: Never thought I'd be so happy not having a roof over my head, eating blueberry pancakes (TOP)!

BOTTOM: Alan's Fried Eggs in Onion Nests

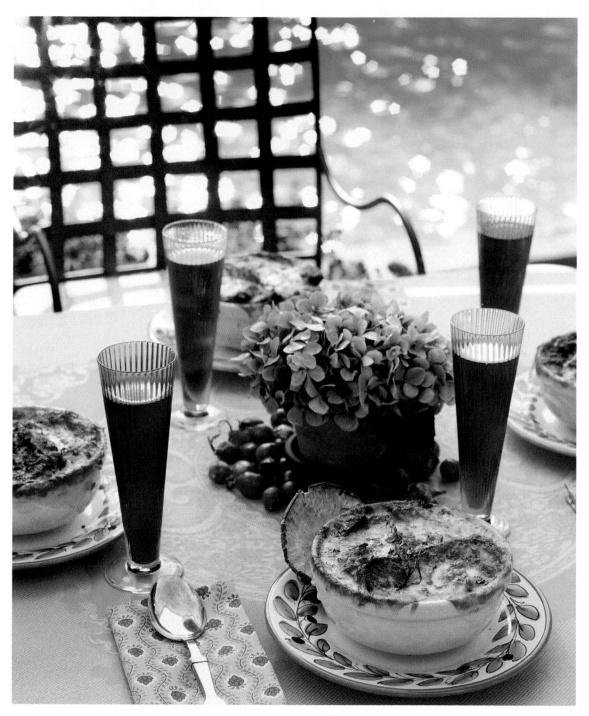

French Onion Soup

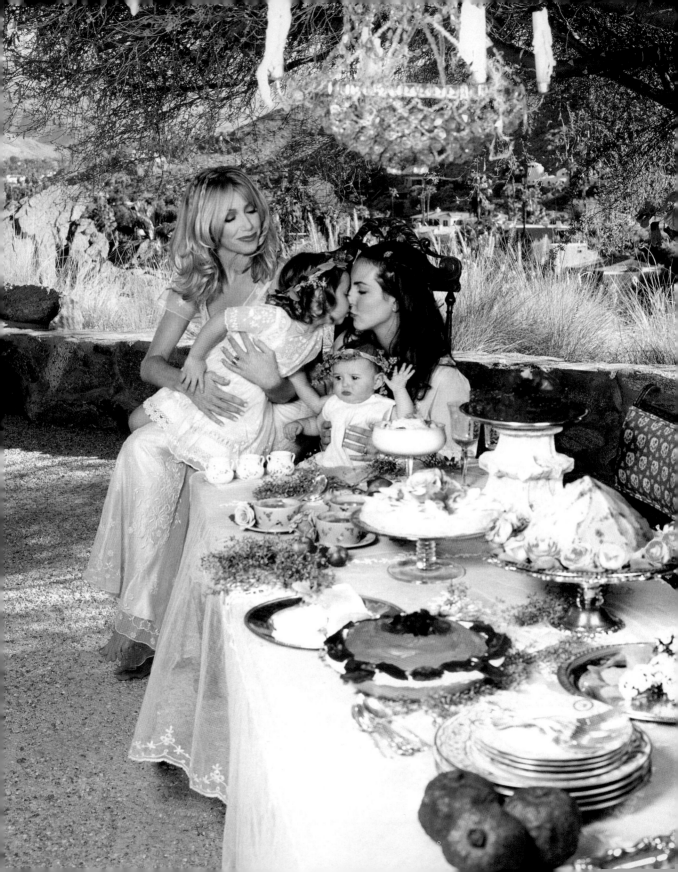

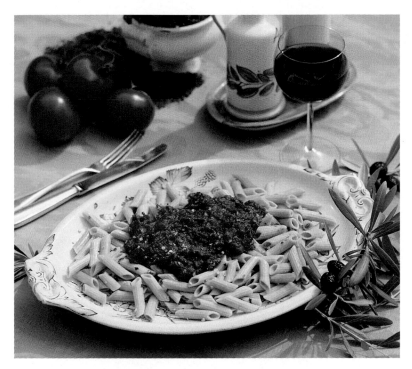

Whole Wheat Penne All'arrabbiata

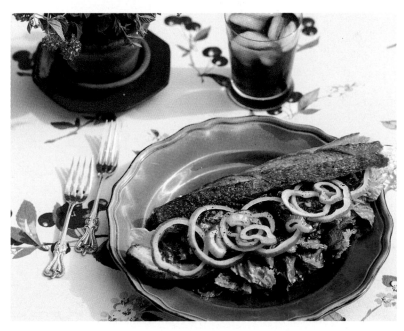

Caesar Salad Sandwich

OPPOSITE: Me and my girls, Camelia, Caroline, and Violet, enjoying a "Somersized" tea party.

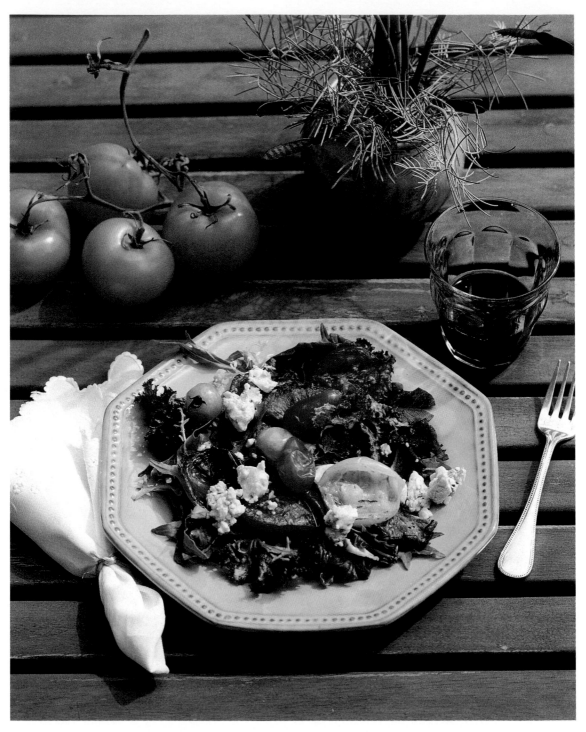

Maytag Blue Cheese and Roasted Vegetable Salad

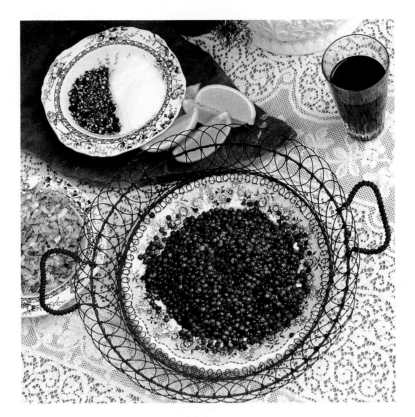

Lentil Salad

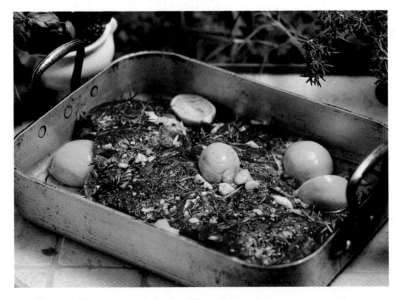

Grilled Butterflied Leg of Lamb marinating in garlic,
olive oil, lemon, and rosemary.

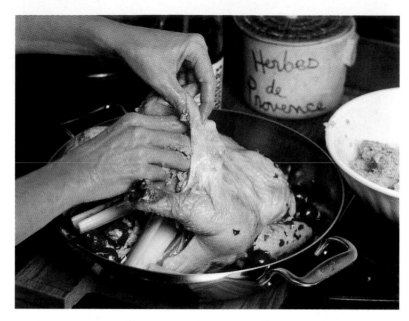

Stuffing under the skin of Farm-Raised Chicken St. Germain Beaupré.

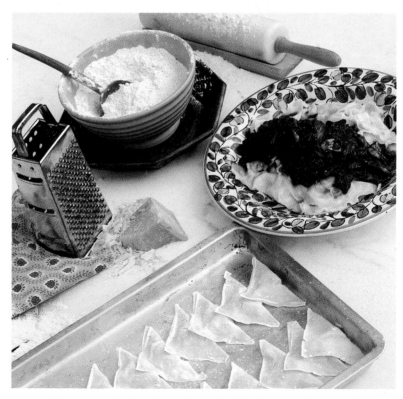

Parsnip Garlic Ravioli with Mushroom Ragout

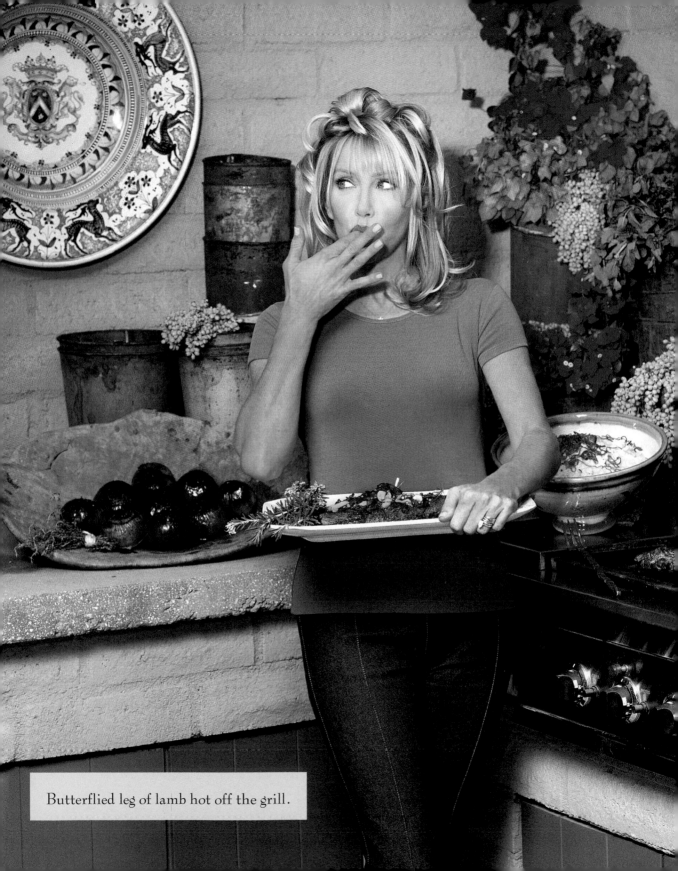
Butterflied leg of lamb hot off the grill.

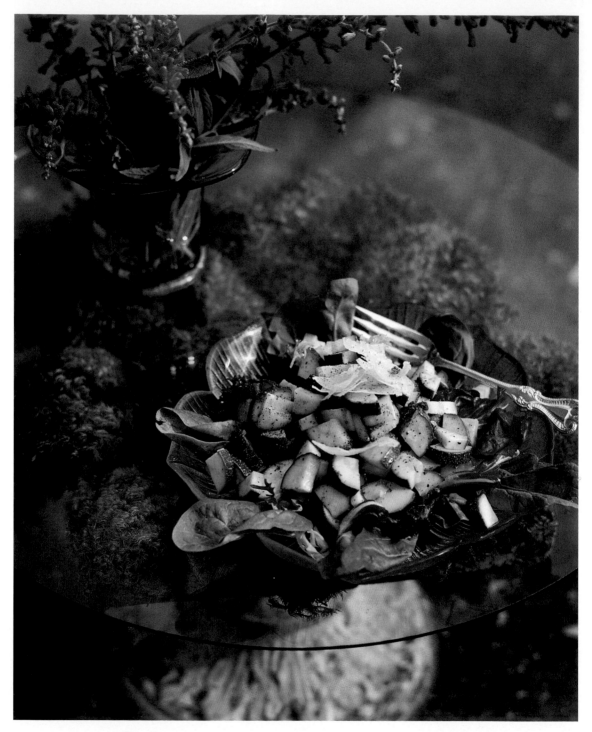

Chopped Raw Zucchini and Parmesan Salad, a wonderful summer lunch.

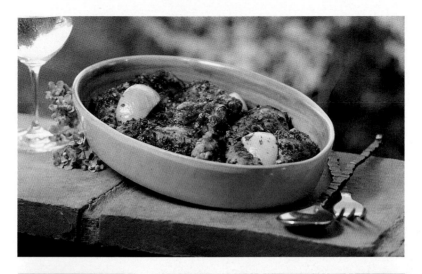

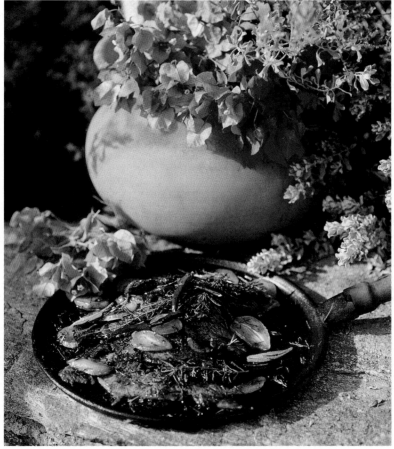

TOP: Crunchy Roasted Lemon Chicken

BOTTOM: Pan-Fried New York Steak with Fried Elephant Garlic

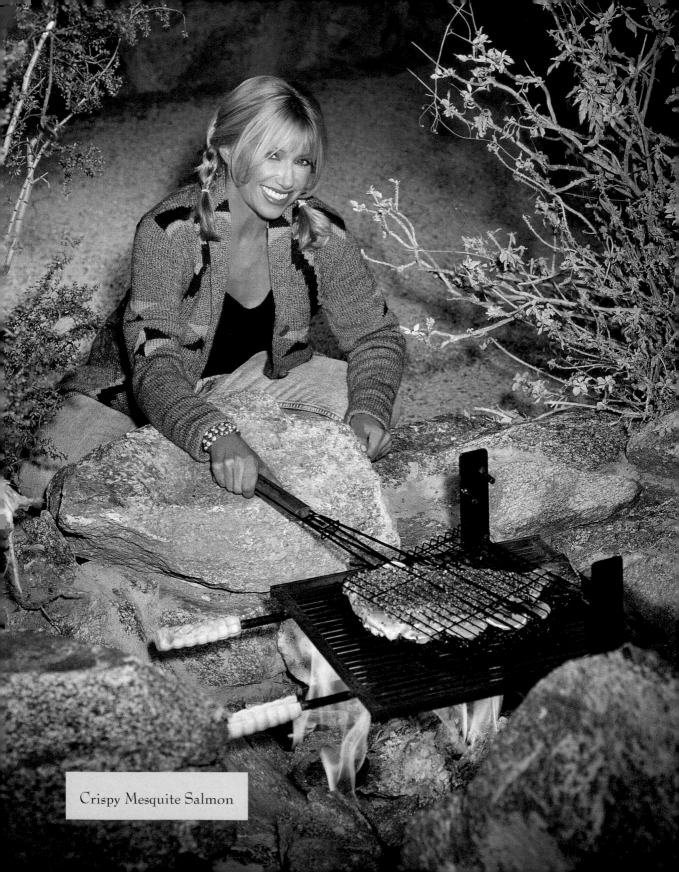

Crispy Mesquite Salmon

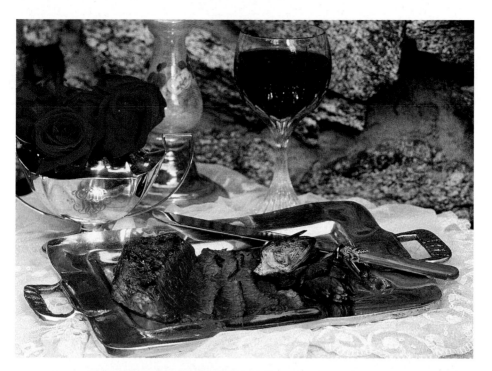

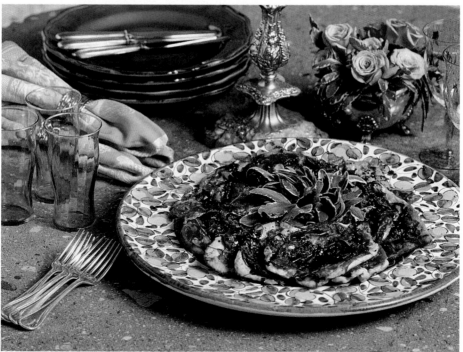

TOP: Rosemary London Broil

BOTTOM: Turkey Prosciutto Piccata with Port Glaze

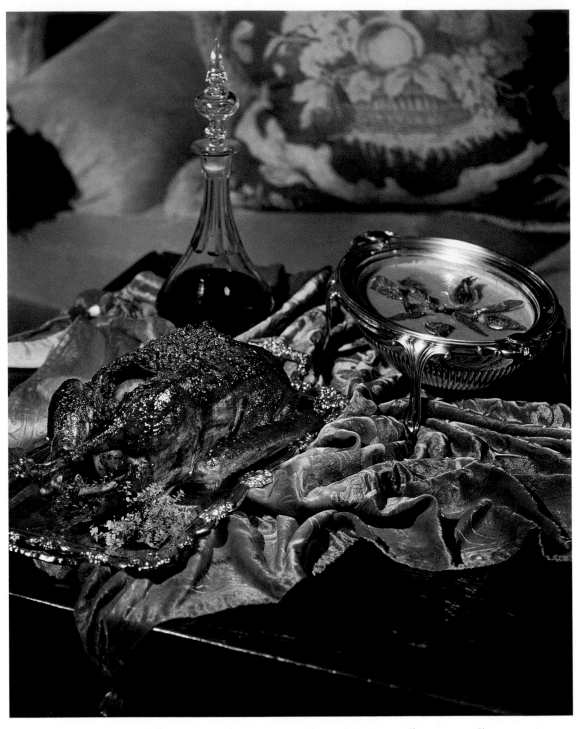

Pumpkin Soup with Roasted Shallots and Sage and Roast Christmas Goose with
Port Glaze, an elegant Christmas meal.

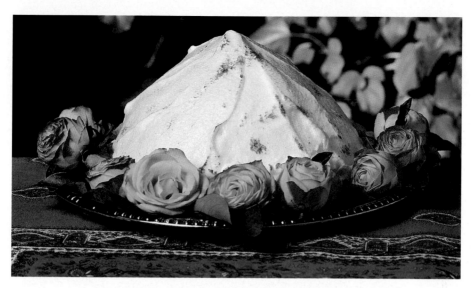

Mountain of Lemon Meringue Pie

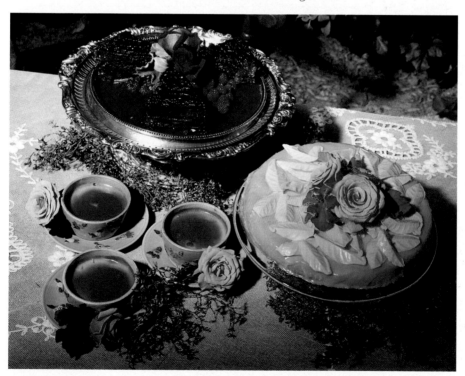

Almond Chocolate Torte with Raspberry Sauce, Decadent White Chocolate Cake,
Ginger Crème Brûlée, Raspberry Crème Brûlée, and Vanilla Crème Brûlée

FOLLOWING PAGE: Stuffed Roast Capon and Endive Salad with Stilton Cheese

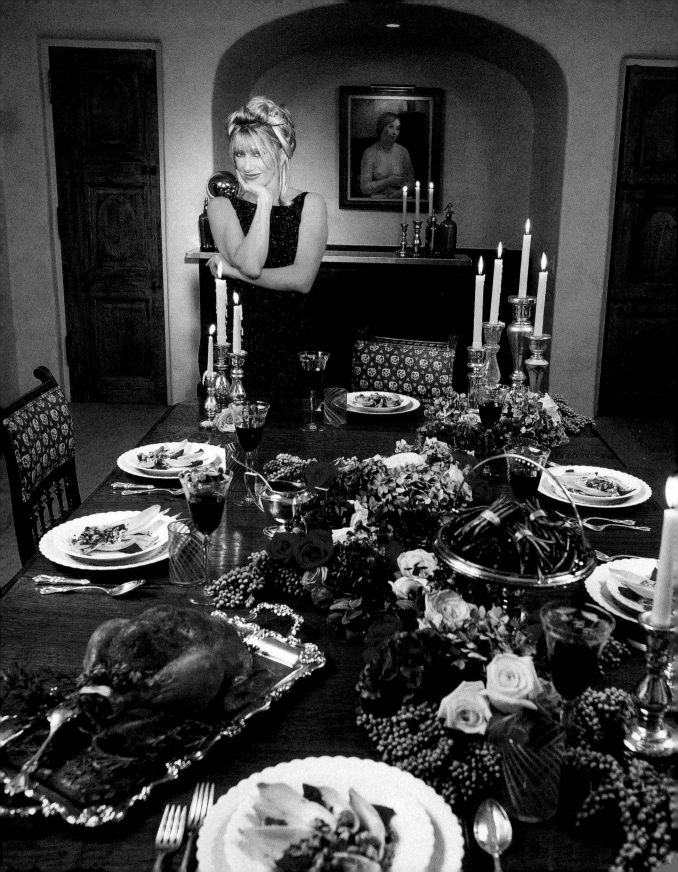

Endive and Radicchio Salad with Stilton Cheese

PROTEINS/FATS AND VEGGIES: LEVEL ONE

SERVES 8

Endive has delicate white leaves, just tipped with pale green on the edges. Radicchio is a small purple Italian cabbage. They make a lovely combination when paired with blue cheese and a balsamic vinaigrette. For Level Two add toasted walnuts.

2 heads of radicchio
4 to 5 heads of endive
8 ounces Stilton cheese, crumbled

BALSAMIC VINAIGRETTE

2 tablespoons balsamic vinegar
Salt and freshly ground black pepper
6 tablespoons extra-virgin olive oil

For each salad, arrange 3 radicchio leaves on the plate. Then fan 4 to 5 endive leaves in a pretty pattern. Crumble the Stilton cheese on top.

For the balsamic vinaigrette, place the vinegar in a mixing cup with salt and pepper to taste. Add the olive oil in a slow stream, constantly whisking until the oil is emulsified. For a tangier dressing, add more balsamic vinegar.

Drizzle the dressing over the salads and serve immediately.

For Level Two
Add one cup of toasted walnuts.

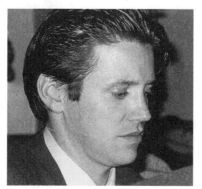

*My son Bruce . . . just because
I like to look at his face.*

Cobb Salad

SERVES 4

Cobb Salad is a Somersizer's best friend at lunch or dinner, in a restaurant or at home. Try my recipe when you feel inspired to make your own. I like to use a variety of lettuces like romaine, red leaf, and butter or red cabbage. Or try the prepackaged salad mix containing 5 or 6 different leaves, including radicchio, curly endive, and Swiss chard.

When chopping the vegetables, meat, and eggs, try to dice them so that all the pieces are uniform in size.

1 pound mixed salad greens
¾ cup Herb Vinaigrette (page 155)
1 small zucchini, diced
4 crisp bacon strips, crumbled
2 large hard-boiled eggs, diced

1 ripe medium tomato, diced
8 ounces crumbled blue cheese (preferably Maytag blue or Roquefort)
¼ pound smoked turkey breast, diced
2 whole green onions, thinly sliced

Place the lettuce in a large salad bowl and toss with the Herb Vinaigrette.

Place the tossed lettuce on 4 large salad plates. Top the greens with vertical rows of meat, cheese, and vegetables. Start by making a vertical row with the zucchini, then a row of bacon, a row of diced egg, a row of diced tomato, a row of cheese, a row of turkey, and a row of green onion slices.

For a tossed Cobb Salad, place all the ingredients in the salad bowl and toss.

Chopped Raw Zucchini and Parmesan Salad

SERVES 6

This was my favorite salad of the summer. We must have eaten it two dozen times. It's fresh. It's crunchy. It's fabulous.

2 pounds green zucchini (use zucchini no larger than 1 inch around for the best taste)
1 pound fresh arugula or Boston lettuce
3 to 4 tablespoons extra-virgin olive oil

2 tablespoons fresh lemon juice, or more to taste
Salt and freshly ground black pepper
1/4 pound Parmesan cheese, in a single piece

Trim the ends off the zucchini and slice into 1/4-inch round pieces. Then coarsely chop into bite-size pieces and set aside.

Wash and dry the arugula or Boston lettuce leaves, discarding any imperfect ones.

In a salad bowl, whisk together the olive oil, lemon juice, and salt and pepper to taste until well combined. Add the zucchini pieces and toss until well coated.

Using a sharp knife or cheese shaver, cut long, paper-thin slices of Parmesan. Place all over the top of the zucchini.

Divide the arugula among 4 serving plates. Spoon the chopped and seasoned zucchini pieces on top of the arugula. Garnish with a few extra shavings of Parmesan. Season with additional salt and pepper and serve immediately.

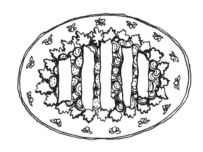

Maytag Blue Cheese and Roasted Vegetable Salad

SERVES 4

The strong flavors of roasted vegetables and Maytag blue cheese give this salad a distinctive flavor. Add a grilled chicken breast and you've got a perfect meal.

2 tablespoons olive oil
1 medium Bermuda onion
1 head of garlic
1 large yellow bell pepper
1 large red bell pepper
2 medium tomatoes

2 heads of Bibb lettuce (about 1 pound), washed, dried, and torn into pieces
3/4 cup Herb Vinaigrette (page 155)
4 tablespoons crumbled Maytag blue cheese (or more if desired)

Preheat the oven to 350°F.

To roast the vegetables, rub a 9 × 12-inch baking dish with 1 tablespoon of olive oil. Cut the onion and garlic in half (around the equator or the middle) and drizzle each side with olive oil. Place the peppers, onion, garlic, and tomatoes in the pan. Reduce the heat to 300°F. and roast the vegetables for 1 hour.

Remove the baking dish from the oven. The vegetables will be brown. Quickly cover with plastic wrap to "steam" the vegetables and set aside for 15 minutes. Remove the plastic wrap. Peel the skin off and remove the seeds from the peppers and tomatoes.

To assemble the salad, toss the lettuce with the Herb Vinaigrette. Arrange on 4 large salad plates. Slice the onion and divide among the salads. Coarsely chop the peppers and tomatoes and divide among the salads. Squeeze the roasted garlic cloves from their skins (at least 3 cloves per salad) and spread over the peppers and onions. Crumble 1 tablespoon of Maytag blue cheese over each salad. Pour a little of the juice from the bottom of the baking pan over the cheese.

Baby Spinach Salad with Vidalia Onions, Sun-Dried Tomatoes, and Goat Cheese

PROTEINS/FATS AND VEGGIES: LEVEL ONE

SERVES 4

Here's a delicious salad with all of my favorite things—baby spinach, sweet onions, sun-dried toma-
toes, goat cheese, and bacon.

8 strips of lean bacon
5 tablespoons olive oil
1 large Vidalia onion, thinly sliced
1 teaspoon crushed garlic
1/4 cup balsamic vinegar
1 teaspoon kosher salt
1 teaspoon freshly ground black pepper

3/4 cup chopped sun-dried tomatoes
3 tablespoons olive oil
1 pound fresh baby or regular spinach,
    destemmed
1 package (10 to 12 ounces) goat cheese,
    sliced into 8 rounds

To fry the bacon, cut the bacon strips into 1-inch pieces. Heat a large skillet over medium-high heat. Add 2 tablespoons of olive oil and heat for a minute or two. Add the bacon and fry until golden brown, gently separating the pieces by stirring with a wooden spoon. Remove the bacon from the skillet and place it on paper towels to absorb the grease.

To make the onions and garlic, pour off all the bacon fat. Place the pan back on the stove over medium heat and add the onions (add a little olive oil, if necessary). Sauté the onions for approximately 10 minutes, until they become golden brown and begin to caramelize. Add the garlic and cook for 1 minute.

Add the vinegar, salt, and pepper, stirring and scraping the pan to get every tasty bit off the bottom. Now add the chopped sun-dried tomatoes and the remaining tablespoons of olive oil, stirring constantly to blend all the flavors.

Divide the cleaned baby spinach among 4 large salad bowls. Place 2 thick round slices of goat cheese on each salad. Sprinkle the bacon pieces on top of the cheese, then place the warm onions and tomatoes over the salad. Drizzle additional hot dressing over the cheese and spinach.

Spinach Salad with Hot Bacon Dressing

SERVES 2

This salad can be prepared in about 15 minutes. It makes a perfect lunch with loads of flavor.

½ pound bacon, cut into 1-inch pieces
2 tablespoons bacon fat
3 tablespoons balsamic vinegar
½ pound fresh spinach leaves, washed and
   dried thoroughly

Salt and freshly ground black pepper
2 large hard-boiled eggs, peeled and
   chopped
10 cherry tomatoes

To cook the bacon, place a large skillet over medium heat. Add the bacon and fry until golden brown, stirring with a wooden spoon to separate the pieces. (If the bacon is burning on the edges, lower the heat. Burned bacon will cause the entire salad to taste burned.) Turn off the heat, then immediately remove the bacon and place on paper towels to absorb the grease.

To make the dressing, pour off all but 2 tablespoons of bacon fat from the hot skillet. Place the skillet back on the stove over medium-high heat. Deglaze the skillet by adding the balsamic vinegar. Heat the vinegar for approximately 1 minute while scraping all the tasty pieces from the bottom of the skillet.

To assemble the salad, place the cleaned spinach in a salad bowl. Toss with the hot bacon dressing and salt and pepper to taste. Divide between 2 plates. Crumble the fried bacon and sprinkle over the salads. Sprinkle on the chopped hard-boiled eggs and garnish with cherry tomatoes.

Hearts of Palm Salad

SERVES 4–6

This perfect little salad is from Urban Epicuria, the "gourmet take-away" in West Hollywood.

1 hothouse cucumber
2 28-ounce cans hearts of palm
2 cups thinly sliced red onions
$\frac{1}{4}$ cup red wine vinegar

$\frac{1}{4}$ cup extra-virgin olive oil
2 tablespoons chopped parsley
2 teaspoons kosher salt
Freshly ground black pepper

Trim the ends of the cucumber and stripe lengthwise with a vegetable peeler. Cut the cucumber in half lengthwise, and then cut each half into $\frac{1}{4}$-inch half-moons.

Drain and rinse the hearts of palm and cut into 1-inch diagonal pieces.

Combine all the ingredients in a bowl and mix gently, being careful not to break up the hearts of palm.

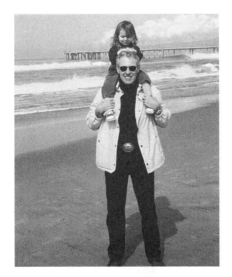

Alan and Camelia.
The children give us so much joy.

Baby Greens with Champagne Vinaigrette

PROTEINS/FATS AND VEGGIES: LEVEL ONE

SERVES 8

Baby greens are tossed in an elegant Champagne vinaigrette for a nice, light salad—ideal for pairing with a rich meal. Pomegranate seeds can be added for a festive touch, making this the perfect holiday salad.

CHAMPAGNE VINAIGRETTE

2 tablespoons Champagne vinegar
1 teaspoon finely chopped fresh basil leaves
Salt and freshly ground black pepper
6 tablespoons extra-virgin olive oil

1 pound mixed baby greens, washed
1/3 cup pomegranate seeds (optional)

For the dressing, place the vinegar in a mixing cup with the basil and salt and pepper to taste. Add the olive oil in a slow stream, constantly whisking until the oil is emulsified.

Toss the washed greens with the vinaigrette. For a perfect Level II meal, garnish each serving with a sprinkle of pomegranate seeds.

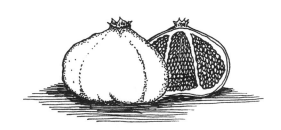

Broccoli and Cauliflower with Lemon-Garlic Vinaigrette

PROTEINS/FATS AND VEGGIES: LEVEL ONE

SERVES 6

After a hard day at work, sometimes Alan and I come home and eat a big bowl of this for dinner. The Lemon-Garlic Vinaigrette is my favorite dressing for salads and vegetables.

1 head of broccoli
1 head of cauliflower

LEMON-GARLIC VINAIGRETTE

2 tablespoons fresh lemon juice
2 garlic cloves, pressed
Salt and freshly ground black pepper
6 tablespoons extra-virgin olive oil

Wash the broccoli and cauliflower. Trim the tough ends off the stalks. Chop the remaining broccoli and cauliflower into large pieces. Put water in the bottom of a large stockpot fitted with a steamer on the stove over high heat. Add the broccoli and cauliflower and steam until tender, 10 to 12 minutes.

To make the vinaigrette, place the lemon juice, garlic, and salt and pepper to taste in a mixing cup. Add the olive oil in a slow stream, constantly whisking until the oil is emulsified. For a tangier dressing, add more lemon juice.

When the broccoli and cauliflower are done, toss in the vinaigrette and serve immediately.

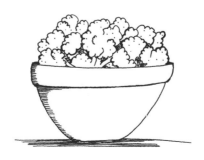

Blue Cheese Vinaigrette with Crudités

PROTEINS/FATS AND VEGGIES: LEVEL ONE

MAKES ABOUT 1½ CUPS VINAIGRETTE

This rich and tangy vinaigrette makes a great salad dressing or dip for crudités (a fancy way to say cut-up vegetables). Use the highest quality blue cheese you can find for the best flavor. I like Maytag blue or a good Roquefort. Make this for a party or keep in your refrigerator for afternoon snacks.

BLUE CHEESE VINAIGRETTE

⅓ cup balsamic vinegar
Salt and freshly ground black pepper
1 cup extra-virgin olive oil
6 ounces blue cheese, crumbled

CRUDITÉS

5 celery stalks, cut into 5-inch-long pieces
10 asparagus stalks, quickly blanched in
    boiling water so they are still a little
    crisp

2 zucchini, cut into strips
1 hothouse cucumber, cut into strips
1 yellow bell pepper, seeded and cut into
    strips
1 red bell pepper, seeded and cut into strips
1 small bag snow peas

To make the vinaigrette, place the vinegar in a mixing cup with salt and pepper to taste. Add the olive oil in a slow stream, constantly whisking until the oil is emulsified. Add the blue cheese and whisk until well combined.

Chill the crudités, then arrange on a beautiful platter with the vinaigrette in the center.

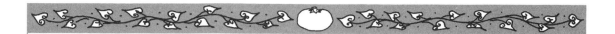

Sauces and Dressings

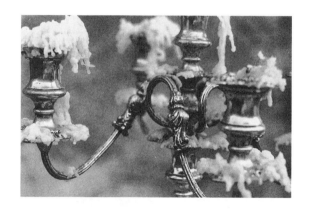

Crème Fraîche

MAKES ABOUT 1 CUP

This tangy sauce has a slightly sour taste. A little dollop is the perfect accent to a bowl of soup or to thicken a sauce. You can buy it premade or use my simple recipe.

1 cup sour cream

1 cup heavy cream

Combine the ingredients in a bowl until slightly thickened. Let sit out at room temperature for several hours to thicken and sour a bit. Then chill and store in the refrigerator. It will keep for approximately a week.

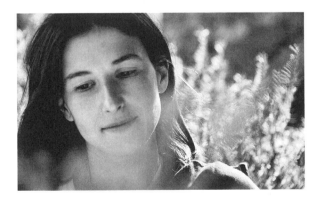

Olivia relaxing at our desert home.

Roasted Vegetable Dip

VEGGIES: LEVEL ONE

MAKES ABOUT 1 QUART

This roasted vegetable dip is one of Ken Brown's biggest sellers at his "gourmet take-away" shop, Urban Epicuria, in West Hollywood. It's made from a puree of roasted vegetables, with a little olive oil, making it perfect for Level One Pro/Fats and Veggies meals. If you want to eat it with Carbos it will create a slight imbalance because of the olive oil, but it's a great choice for Level Two. Try it as a dip with cut-up vegetables, a sandwich spread on whole-grain bread, or a dipping sauce with whole-wheat pita. Thanks for sharing this and your other great recipes, Ken!

1 medium eggplant, peeled and cut into chunks
¼ cup olive oil
2 cups diced yellow onions
2 garlic cloves, chopped
1 tablespoon dried basil
1 tablespoon dried oregano
1 teaspoon ground cumin
1 tablespoon sweet paprika
1 to 2 roasted red bell peppers, roughly chopped
1 tablespoon fresh lemon juice
Salt and freshly ground black pepper

Before assembling your ingredients, salt the eggplant and let it drain in a colander for 30 minutes. Squeeze out any excess liquid and pat dry.

Heat the olive oil in a medium sauté pan and add the eggplant and onions.

When the vegetables are soft, add the garlic, basil, oregano, cumin, and paprika and cook 5 minutes, or until the aromas are released.

Remove from the heat, and add the roasted peppers.

Transfer the mixture to a food processor and blend until smooth. Finish with the lemon juice and salt and pepper to taste.

Tomatillo Salsa

VEGGIES: LEVEL ONE

MAKES ABOUT 1½ CUPS

Tomatillos are small green Mexican tomatoes that make a mild green salsa. If you cannot find them, substitute unripe green tomatoes.

15 tomatillos, husks removed, quartered
1 bunch of cilantro
5 garlic cloves

3 serrano chilies
1 teaspoon salt
Juice of 1 lime

Blend all the ingredients in a food processor or a blender until pureed.

Pico de Gallo

VEGGIES: LEVEL ONE

MAKES ABOUT 2 CUPS

Caroline makes the best salsa. Whenever she asks what she can bring to our house for dinner, I say, "Your fabulous salsa." I love it on chicken breasts or steaks. And it's great on my Twelve-Hour Roast Pork (page 222). Increase the amount of serranos if you like your salsa hotter.

4 ripe medium tomatoes, diced
½ medium cucumber, diced
1 bunch of cilantro, coarsely chopped
1 medium red onion, diced

2 serrano chilies, finely chopped, with
  seeds
1 garlic clove, minced
Juice of 2 limes

Gently combine all the ingredients in a nonmetallic bowl and set aside for the flavors to combine, about 30 minutes. Do not refrigerate or the tomatoes will get mushy.

Herb Vinaigrette

PROTEINS/FATS: LEVEL ONE

MAKES ABOUT 3/4 CUP

2 tablespoons red wine vinegar
1 garlic clove, pressed
2 teaspoons whole-grain mustard
1 teaspoon dried dill weed

1 teaspoon dried thyme
Salt and freshly ground black pepper
6 tablespoons extra-virgin olive oil

Whisk together all the ingredients except the olive oil. Add the oil in a slow stream, whisking constantly until the oil is emulsified. For a tangier dressing, add more vinegar.

Roasted Red Pepper Vinaigrette

PROTEINS/FATS AND VEGGIES: LEVEL ONE

MAKES ABOUT 1 CUP

This makes a great dressing for salads or dip for vegetables. If you have time to roast your own peppers, try my recipe (EGLW, page 81). If not, jarred peppers work beautifully.

1 cup roasted red peppers
¼ cup extra-virgin olive oil
1 tablespoon fresh lemon juice
4 fresh basil leaves, chopped

1 teaspoon dried oregano
1 teaspoon minced fresh garlic
Salt and freshly ground black pepper

Place the roasted peppers, olive oil, lemon juice, basil, oregano, and garlic in the blender. Puree until smooth. Season with salt and pepper.

Creole Butter

MAKES ABOUT 1 POUND

I like to keep this tasty butter in the freezer. I melt it on seafood just off the grill, broiled fish, or steaks.

1 tablespoon olive oil
1 shallot, minced
3 garlic cloves, minced
1 pound (4 sticks) butter, softened
1 teaspoon cayenne

1 teaspoon white pepper
2 teaspoons garlic salt
5 thyme sprigs, stems removed
1 teaspoon picante sauce

Place a small skillet over medium heat. Add the olive oil and the shallot. Sauté the shallot until it is tender and translucent. And the garlic and sauté 1 minute more. Remove from the heat and let cool.

Place the shallot and garlic with the remaining ingredients in a mixing bowl and blend together to incorporate the flavors of the garlic and shallot into the softened butter. Cover and freeze until needed.

Lemon Pepper Marinade

MAKES ABOUT 2 CUPS

This is a great marinade for chicken and fish. I also use it as a sauce and basting liquid.

1 tablespoon black peppercorns
¼ cup fresh lemon juice
1 8-ounce can chicken broth
1 tablespoon tarragon or white wine
    vinegar

¾ cup extra-virgin olive oil
3 fresh garlic cloves, minced

Place the peppercorns in a plastic bag and seal. Pound with a mallet or the bottom of a frying pan to crack the peppercorns.

Place the peppercorns and all the remaining ingredients in a blender and mix until well combined.

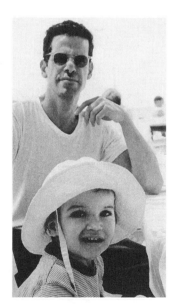

Stephen and our adorable grandson.

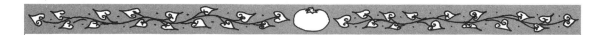

Pasta

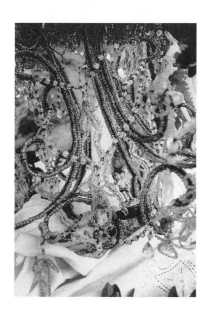

Whole-Grain Pasta with Candied Tomato Sauce

CARBOS AND VEGGIES: LEVEL ONE

SERVES 4

I received so many letters from people who love my Candied Tomatoes from Eat Great, Lose Weight. *Here's a recipe for pasta sauce made from the Candied Tomatoes. If you make the tomatoes without oil, you can use this sauce on your favorite whole-grain pasta during Level One. If you make them with oil, then the sauce becomes a Pro/Fats and Veggies and can be combined with any of the foods from that group, or it can be used on Level Two with whole-grain pasta.*

CANDIED TOMATOES

24 ripe tomatoes
Salt
Fresh thyme, chopped

1 pound whole-grain pasta
5 basil leaves, chopped

Preheat the oven to 325°F.

Slice the tomatoes in half, crosswise. Place the tomatoes on a baking sheet, cut side up. Sprinkle with salt and thyme. Bake for 2 to 3 hours until the tomatoes are wrinkled on the outside, crusty on the bottom, but still somewhat moist in the center.

Place the tomatoes in a food processor and puree until smooth (or you can put the tomatoes in a mixing bowl and blend with an electric mixer). If the sauce is too thick, thin it with a little pasta water until it reaches the desired consistency.

In a large pot, bring salted water to a rolling boil. Cook the pasta according to package instructions until al dente (cooked through but not mushy). Drain the pasta in a colander, reserving a little of the pasta water to use in the sauce.

Top the pasta with the sauce. Garnish with basil leaves and serve immediately.

For Level Two
Drizzle olive oil over the tomatoes before you put them in the oven. And you may sprinkle a little Parmesan cheese over the top, if you like.

Whole-Wheat Penne All'arrabbiata

SERVES 4

This is a simple, quick, tasty Level One pasta meal. Arrabiata means spicy tomato sauce. You'll love the flavor. Serve with a steamed green vegetable, such as broccoli or spinach.

2 1-pound, 12-ounce cans crushed Italian
   plum tomatoes with juice
6 garlic cloves, peeled and minced
Salt
2 teaspoons hot red pepper flakes (or more,
   if desired)

1 pound whole-wheat penne
1/2 teaspoon dried oregano
10 fresh basil leaves, cut into julienne

Place a large skillet over medium-high heat. Add a couple of tablespoons of tomato juice from the canned tomatoes. Add the garlic and sauté in the tomato juice until soft, 7 to 10 minutes. Add the remaining tomatoes and salt to taste and bring to a boil. Lower the heat to simmer, add the pepper flakes, and cook for 20 to 25 minutes. The sauce will reduce and thicken.

In another large stockpot, bring salted water to a rolling boil. Add the penne. Cook until al dente (cooked through but not mushy) for 8 to 10 minutes. Do not overcook. Drain in a colander, reserving 1/2

cup of the pasta water. (This is an important step that good Italian cooks know about. The pasta water thickens the sauce.)

Put the penne, pasta water, and tomato sauce back into a large soup pot and toss until each piece is well coated. Add the oregano and basil. Adjust the seasonings. Serve immediately.

For Level Two
Sauté the garlic in 1/4 cup olive oil instead of the tomato juice. Also, you may toss the penne with freshly grated Parmesan cheese.

Whole-Wheat Spaghetti with Broccoli

CARBOS AND VEGGIES: LEVEL ONE

SERVES 4

1 pound whole-wheat spaghetti
3 garlic cloves, peeled and minced
1 pound broccoli, steamed

1 cup vegetable stock (page 126)
Salt and freshly ground black pepper
Pinch of hot red pepper flakes (optional)

On the stovetop, bring a large stockpot of salted water to a rolling boil. Add the spaghetti and cook until al dente, 7 to 10 minutes, reserving a little pasta water.

While the spaghetti is cooking, heat a large skillet on another burner over medium heat. When hot, add about ¼ cup of the pasta water and the garlic. Cook until soft, 7 to 10 minutes. Add the cooked broccoli, vegetable stock, and salt and pepper to taste. Simmer for 5 minutes. Set aside.

When the spaghetti is cooked, drain it in a colander. Reheat the broccoli mixture over medium-high heat and add the spaghetti. Toss together for 1 minute. Adjust the seasonings. Add hot red pepper flakes if you prefer this dish spicy.

Serve immediately.

For Level Two
Sauté the garlic in ¼ cup olive oil instead of the pasta water. And use chicken stock (pages 123 and 125) instead of the vegetable stock for more flavor. Top with Parmesan cheese, if you like.

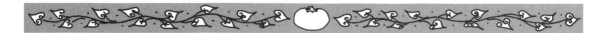

Vegetables and Side Dishes

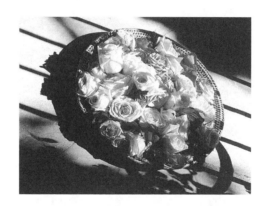

Stuffed Mushrooms

PROTEINS/FATS AND VEGGIES: LEVEL ONE

MAKES ABOUT 12

Need a great little appetizer? Look no further. These stuffed mushrooms are simple and delicious. Make plenty! They're also great with a salad for a light lunch, or to serve alongside your favorite meat, poultry, or fish. I make them with lemon thyme that grows in my garden. You can substitute any herb, such as parsley or tarragon.

1 pound mushrooms
4 tablespoons (½ stick) butter
4 shallots, finely chopped
1 tablespoon chopped lemon thyme (or parsley or tarragon)

Salt and freshly ground black pepper
½ cup grated Parmesan cheese
2 tablespoons olive oil
¼–½ cup dry white wine

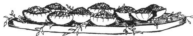

The mushroom stems will be used as part of the stuffing. Begin by trimming the very end off the mushroom stems. Then carefully pull the stems off the mushrooms. Finely chop the mushroom stems. Select the 12 largest mushroom caps and set aside. Thinly slice the remaining mushrooms, then chop.

Melt the butter in a large skillet over medium heat. Add the shallots and sauté until golden, about 5 minutes. Add the mushroom stems, the chopped mushrooms, the lemon thyme, and salt and pepper to taste. Sauté until the mushrooms are browned and crusty, about 10 minutes. Add the white wine and let it cook off for about 3 minutes, scraping the bits from the bottom of the pan to release the flavor. Remove from the heat.

Preheat the broiler.

Place the mushroom mixture in a mixing bowl with half of the Parmesan cheese (¼ cup). Stir until well combined.

Lightly rub the reserved mushroom caps with the olive oil and place on a cookie sheet with the cavity side up. Fill each cavity with a heaping mound of the mushroom stuffing. Sprinkle the remaining ¼ cup Parmesan over the top of the stuffed mushrooms.

Place the cookie sheet under the broiler for approximately 5 minutes.

Keep a close eye on them. You want the cheese to be bubbly and the mushroom caps to get a little brown. If your broiler is very hot the cheese may start to burn before the mushroom caps are cooked. In that case, lower the rack to allow the mushrooms to cook longer without burning the tops. Transfer to a platter and serve sizzling hot.

Mushroom-Shallot Dressing

PROTEINS/FATS AND VEGGIES: LEVEL ONE

SERVES 6

When it comes to side dishes for turkey or chicken, a stuffing gets cooked inside the cavity, whereas a dressing is cooked separately and served on the side. This one is perfect with my Farm-Raised Chicken St. Germain Beaupré (page 195).

2 tablespoons olive oil
10 whole shallots, minced
1 pound mushrooms (any kind or a
    mixture), chopped
Salt and freshly ground black pepper

2 tablespoons fresh tarragon leaves or 1
    tablespoon dried
1/2 cup dry white wine
2 tablespoons (1/4 stick) unsalted butter

Heat a skillet over medium heat. Add the olive oil. When the oil is just getting hot, add the shallots, stirring constantly so they brown but do not burn, 5 to 7 minutes. When the shallots are beginning to brown, add the mushrooms, turning often until they become soft and crusty on the edges, 10 to 15 minutes. Season with salt and pepper and tarragon.

Turn the heat up to high and add the white wine. Let the wine cook off for a couple of minutes, scraping the bits from the bottom of the pan. Then lower the heat and simmer for another 10 minutes. Turn off the heat and add the butter, 1 tablespoon at a time, stirring until the butter is melted and the mushrooms are coated.

Asian Braised String Beans

SERVES 6

There is a Szechuan restaurant near our home where we love the braised string beans. They are cooked in a very hot wok until the skin bubbles. The result is crispy green beans with lots of garlic, ginger, and soy sauce. This recipe also works great with asparagus.

2 tablespoons peanut oil
2 tablespoons minced garlic
1 tablespoon grated fresh ginger

1 pound string beans, ends trimmed
¼ teaspoon hot red pepper flakes (optional)
¼ cup soy sauce

Heat a wok over high heat. Add the peanut oil and heat for a minute or two. Add the garlic and ginger and sauté for 1 to 2 minutes. Add the string beans and red pepper flakes, if using, and sauté for approx-imately 5 minutes, until the skin bubbles. The beans should be tender, but still a little crispy. Add the soy sauce and sauté for another 30 seconds or so. Serve immedi-ately.

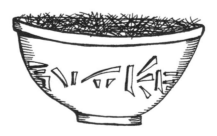

Summer Stir-Fry

PROTEINS/FATS AND VEGGIES: LEVEL ONE

SERVES 4

The key to stir-frying is keeping the wok or pan very hot. Always stir-fry in small batches to accomplish this.

1 to 3 tablespoons peanut oil
2 yellow summer squash, cut into julienne
2 small zucchini, cut into julienne
1 leek, cut into julienne
1 bunch of asparagus, cut into bite-size
   pieces

2 tablespoons soy sauce
Juice of ½ lemon
Hot chili oil to taste

Heat a wok over high heat. Add 1 tablespoon of the oil and the yellow squash, stirring constantly for about 2 minutes, or until tender and still a little crunchy. Remove the squash and set aside. Add the zucchini and cook for about 2 minutes. Add more oil as needed. Remove and set aside. Repeat with the leek, then the asparagus.

Place all the vegetables back in the wok with the soy sauce and lemon juice. Toss until well coated. Remove from the heat and serve immediately. Add a couple dishes of hot chili oil if you want.

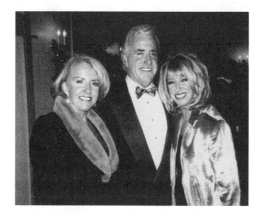

My sister Maureen Gilmartin, my big brother Dan Mahoney, and me at a family party.

Grilled Vegetable Tower

SERVES 4

There's nothing like a stack of grilled vegetables. Then top it off with crumbled feta cheese and a reduction of balsamic vinegar. Delicious. Try this with the Persian Kabobs (page 209). For a Carbos and Veggies meal, eliminate the oil and cheese, then stack the vegetables on crusty whole-grain bread.

2 medium zucchini, sliced on the diagonal into 1/2-inch slices
1 red onion, cut into 1/2-inch rings
1 red bell pepper, quartered and seeded
1 yellow bell pepper, quartered and seeded
1 fennel bulb, cut into 1/2-inch slices

1 carton cherry tomatoes
1 eggplant, sliced into 1/2-inch-thick slices
Olive oil
Salt and freshly ground black pepper
1/2 cup balsamic vinegar
8 ounces feta cheese, crumbled

Preheat the grill to medium-high heat.

Brush all the vegetables with a little olive oil. Season with salt and pepper. Place as many vegetables on the grill as will fit at one time. The onions, pepper, and fennel will take the longest. Remove the vegetables as they become tender. You want them to have char marks, but not to be burned.

Place the vinegar in a small saucepan over high heat. Reduce by half or more, until thickened and syrupy.

Stack the grilled vegetables into 4 towers. Start with a slice of eggplant, then the onions, then the red pepper, the fennel, the yellow pepper, then the zucchini. (Stack another layer high, if you wish, with the leftover vegetables.) Strew the tomatoes around the plate. Crumble the feta cheese over the top. Drizzle the hot balsamic vinegar over the top and serve.

Celery Root Puree with Olive Oil and Crispy Fried Onions

PROTEINS/FATS AND VEGGIES: LEVEL ONE

SERVES 4 TO 6

In Eat Great, Lose Weight, *I included a delicious recipe for celery root pureed with butter and cream. In this version I don't use any dairy, just olive oil. Then I top it with crispy fried onions. It may even be better than the original.*

3 large celery roots
$\frac{1}{3}$ cup olive oil
Salt and freshly ground black pepper

FRIED ONIONS

1 tablespoon olive oil
1 onion, thinly sliced

In a large pot fitted with a steamer and a lid, bring to a boil about 5 cups of water.

Chop off the roots and peel off the outside layer of skin from the celery roots, being careful to remove all the brown. Cut each celery root into 12 pieces and place the pieces in the steamer. Steam until very soft when poked with a fork, about 20 minutes.

Transfer the celery root to a food processor. Add the olive oil and puree until smooth. (If you don't have a food processor, you can use an electric mixer.) Add additional olive oil to achieve the desired consistency. Sprinkle with salt and pepper.

While the celery root is simmering, place the olive oil in a saucepan over medium heat to make the fried onions. When the oil is hot, place the sliced onion into the pan. Keep stirring while the onion starts to brown. Continue cooking until the onion is brown and crispy. Remove and drain on paper towels.

Serve the celery root with crispy fried onions on top.

Fried Rice with Shiitake Mushrooms
CARBOS AND VEGGIES: LEVEL ONE

SERVES 4

When you need a Carbo fix, this fried rice is fabulous.

1 shallot, minced
¼ cup uncooked wild rice
¼ cup uncooked brown rice
¼ cup dried shiitake mushrooms

2 cups vegetable stock (page 126)
1 tablespoon balsamic vinegar
½ cup frozen baby peas

Soak the dried mushrooms in 2 cups of warm water. Place a large skillet over medium-high heat with 2 tablespoons of water. Add the shallot and sauté until tender. Add the rices and stir together. Drain the mushrooms and coarsely chop. Then add to the vegetable stock. Bring to a boil, then lower the heat and cover. Simmer for 25 minutes.

Add the vinegar and peas. Cover and simmer for another 5 minutes.

Zucchini and Summer Squash Ribbons
PROTEINS/FATS AND VEGGIES: LEVEL ONE

SERVES 4

In this recipe I cut the squash into long thin ribbons for a beautiful presentation.

2 medium zucchini
2 medium Italian yellow summer squash
1 tablespoon butter

1 teaspoon dried dill weed
Salt and freshly ground black pepper
1 tablespoon fresh lemon juice

Wash and dry the squash. With a vegetable peeler or mandoline, slice the squash lengthwise into long thin ribbons.

Heat the butter in a large skillet. Add the ribbons of squash and dill. Toss around to cover with the hot butter. Be careful not to overcook. The squash should just start to get limp, 3 to 4 minutes. Season with salt and pepper and the lemon juice.

Sautéed Spinach with Garlic and Olive Oil

PROTEINS/FATS AND VEGGIES: LEVEL ONE

SERVES 2

This is a great side dish for your favorite Italian main courses. Look for bags of prewashed spinach to save on prep time.

2 tablespoons olive oil
2 garlic cloves, peeled
1 pound fresh spinach leaves, washed
    thoroughly and drained

Salt and freshly ground black pepper

To a hot skillet, add the olive oil and the peeled garlic. Sauté the garlic for 5 minutes, until it begins to brown and get soft.

Add the spinach to the pan and toss in the hot oil until each piece is coated and just wilted. Season with salt and pepper. Serve immediately.

Broccoli Rabe with Garlic and Hot Pepper

PROTEINS/FATS AND VEGGIES: LEVEL ONE

SERVES 4

This is spicy, fresh, and delicious! I love it with chicken piccata or grilled fish.

Kosher salt
1 bundle of broccoli rabe
3 tablespoons olive oil
2 garlic cloves, thinly sliced

1 teaspoon crushed red pepper flakes
Freshly ground black pepper
2 tablespoons fresh lemon juice

In a large saucepan, bring 2 quarts of salted water to a boil.

Wash the broccoli rabe, cut off the bottom, and remove any yellow leaves. Cut into 2-inch pieces. Place the broccoli rabe into the boiling water and cook until slightly tender. Drain.

Wipe out the pan and place it back on the stove over medium heat. Add the olive oil. Add the garlic and red pepper flakes. Sauté until the garlic turns light golden brown. Add the broccoli rabe and toss well.

Season with more salt, pepper to taste, and the lemon juice.

Artichokes with Roasted Red Pepper Vinaigrette

SERVES 2

This beautiful artichoke salad makes a great starter for company. Try adding crabmeat for an entrée.

2 medium artichokes
Juice of ½ lemon
2 teaspoons vegetable oil
3 cups vegetable or chicken stock (pages 126 or 123 and 125)

1 head of radicchio
⅓ cup Roasted Red Pepper Vinaigrette (page 155)
Salt and freshly ground black pepper
Chopped parsley

To make the artichokes, place the artichokes, on their sides, on a cutting board. With a sharp knife, cut off the stem and about 2 inches of the top. Using scissors, trim off the remaining sharp leaf tips.

In a large skillet, sit the artichokes bottom side down. Drizzle with the lemon juice and oil. Pour the stock into the skillet, cover, and cook over medium heat for 25 minutes, keeping an eye on the liquid level.

Do not let the pan dry out. When they are done, you will be able to pull off any leaf easily.

While the artichokes are cooking, wash the radicchio and arrange on 2 plates.

When the artichokes are done, cut them in half and serve with Roasted Red Pepper Vinaigrette drizzled over the top. Season with salt and pepper. Garnish with chopped parsley. The dish can be served hot or cold.

Tuscan Artichoke Pâté

MAKES ABOUT 2 CUPS

This recipe comes from my daughter-in-law, Caroline. She's a wonder in the kitchen. Artichoke pâté is decadent and delicious. It's best when made with fresh artichoke bottoms, but canned will work if you do not have time or if artichokes are not in season. It makes the perfect complement to grilled or roasted meats. And it's great for antipasto spreads with Roasted Peppers and Grilled Bread (EGLW, page 81) and Candied Tomatoes (EGLW, page 76).

2 12-ounce cans artichoke bottoms
2 cups chicken stock (pages 123 and 125)
¼ cup fresh lemon juice

1 tablespoon extra-virgin olive oil
Sea salt
Freshly ground black pepper

Drain the artichoke bottoms and place in a saucepan with the chicken stock and fresh lemon juice. Simmer gently for about 10 minutes. Remove the artichokes from the pan and place in a blender or food processor. Add the olive oil, a little sea salt, and pepper to taste. Blend until smooth and well combined.

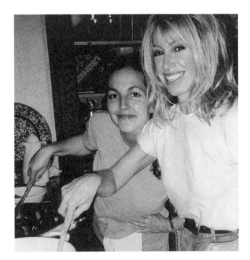

Caroline and I often cook together.

Grilled Artichokes

SERVES 4

My son Bruce's favorite food is the artichoke. In Eat Great, Lose Weight, *I had a couple of recipes, one for steaming and one for frying. Now I've brought them to the grill. Surprise, surprise . . . Bruce loves them.*

4 medium artichokes
$\frac{1}{4}$ cup olive oil
4 garlic cloves
8 fresh thyme sprigs
1 tablespoon kosher salt
1 large lemon, quartered

FOR BASTING

2 tablespoons olive oil
Salt and freshly ground pepper

GARNISH

2 lemons, halved

Preheat the grill to medium-high heat.

In a stockpot, bring 1 quart of water to a boil.

Trim the stems of the artichokes. Cut each in half lengthwise. With the tip of a knife, scrape out the choke (the sharp little hairs). Rinse well. Place the artichoke halves, along with the olive oil, garlic, thyme, salt, and quartered lemon, into the boiling water and lower the heat. Simmer for 20 minutes, or until tender.

Drain the artichokes. Place the artichoke halves on the hot grill and let them char a little, turning frequently, for about 5 minutes on each side. Just before removing, baste them with olive oil. Season with salt and pepper and serve with lemon wedges.

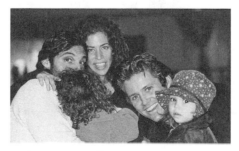

Our kids all hang out together.

Spaghetti Squash

PROTEINS/FATS AND VEGGIES: LEVEL ONE

SERVES 4

Spaghetti squash is an overlooked vegetable worth noting . . . and eating!

1 medium spaghetti squash
Salt and freshly ground pepper

3 tablespoons unsalted butter
1 tablespoon vegetable oil

Slice the squash in half, lengthwise.

Place the slices on an oiled baking sheet, cut side down. Cook 40 to 60 minutes or until a fork easily pierces the flesh. When cooked, scoop out the flesh into a bowl and discard the skin. Separate the flesh into strands. Toss with butter, salt, and pepper to taste.

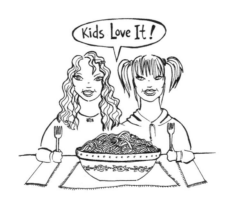

Grilled Radicchio

SERVES 4

Radicchio is an Italian red cabbage with a firm texture and slightly bitter flavor. When grilled with olive oil and balsamic vinegar, it becomes slightly charred and incredibly sweet. This is great with Balsamic Roast Chicken (page 197), Marinated Grilled Butterflied Leg of Lamb (page 219), and most roasted or grilled meats.

2 heads of radicchio
¼ cup olive oil

2 tablespoons balsamic vinegar
Sea salt and freshly ground black pepper

Preheat the grill to medium-high heat.

Slice the radicchio in half lengthwise. Rinse and pat it dry.

Combine the olive oil, balsamic vinegar, and salt and pepper to taste in a bowl. Rub the oil mixture over the halved radicchio pieces.

Place on a hot grill for 3 to 5 minutes on each side. The radicchio is done when it's warm with a few char marks but still has a little crunch. Serve immediately.

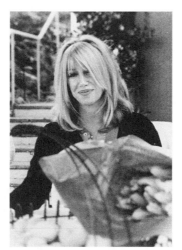

Setting the table for another spectacular family luncheon.

Roasted Tomatoes with Rosemary and Garlic

SERVES 4

Oh, the versatile tomato! These little yummies are roasted with rosemary and garlic—the perfect side dish to meat, poultry, or fish.

2 tablespoons olive oil
4 plum tomatoes, halved lengthwise
Salt and freshly ground black pepper
2 garlic cloves, thinly sliced into 16 slices

1 tablespoon chopped fresh rosemary (or 2 teaspoons dried rosemary)
1 tablespoon grated Parmesan cheese
2 tablespoons chopped parsley

Preheat the oven to 350° F.

Brush a baking sheet with olive oil and place the tomatoes on it, cut side up. Brush the tomatoes with the remaining oil and sprinkle with salt and pepper.

With a paring knife, make 2 slits in each tomato and stuff each with a slice of garlic. Sprinkle the rosemary and cheese over the top and place in the oven for 45 minutes.

Garnish with the parsley.

Baked Caramelized Onions

PROTEINS/FATS AND VEGGIES: LEVEL ONE

SERVES 8

These onions are my favorite creation of the year! It may seem like a lot of work for an onion, but you won't believe how great they are . . . perhaps my favorite recipe in the book. I prefer red onions, but Vidalia or Maui onions will also work well. The balsamic vinegar and wine sauce cooks down to a sweet syrup.

8 small onions (red, Maui, or Vidalia)
4 garlic cloves
8 tablespoons (1 stick) unsalted butter
1 bunch of thyme

Salt and freshly ground black pepper
1½ cups balsamic vinegar
1½ cups red wine

Preheat the oven to 350°F.

To prepare the onions, remove the skins from the onions. Trim the base of each onion so they can sit upright without falling over. Place the onions on a cutting board and cut a deep cross on the top of each onion by slicing down from the top about halfway down the height of the onion. With an apple corer or the head of a potato peeler, carve out a small piece of the center of each onion, again starting from the top. You want to create a cavity large enough to fill with the garlic cloves and butter. Be careful not to carve all the way through to the bottom of the onion or the butter will run out.

To prepare the filling, cut each garlic clove into 4 slivers, creating 16 slivers. In a small dish, combine the butter and fresh thyme until the butter is softened.

To stuff the onions, put 2 slivers of garlic and 1 tablespoon of the butter-thyme mixture into the cavity of each onion. Place the onions in a roasting pan and season with salt and pepper. Drizzle half of the balsamic vinegar and half of the red wine over the onions.

Bake for 1 hour, or until the onions are soft. Then reduce the oven temperature to 300°F. Continue to cook for 1 hour more, basting frequently with the pan juices. When the juices start drying up, add the remaining balsamic vinegar and red wine. The onions are ready when they look slightly crispy and caramelized on the outside edges and are soft on the inside. The pan juices will be thick and caramelized.

To serve, spoon the thick sauce over each onion.

Fennel and Leeks au Gratin

PROTEINS/FATS AND VEGGIES: LEVEL ONE

SERVES 4

When you're craving potatoes, this au gratin does the trick. It's creamy, rich, and delicious. The key to this dish is a good-quality Parmesan cheese. My favorite is Parmigiano-Reggiano. I love this as a side dish to chicken or fish. It also makes a nice light meal as an entrée, served with my Candied Tomatoes (EGLW, page 76).

1 tablespoon olive oil
4 medium fennel bulbs
4 medium leeks
6 tablespoons (¾ stick) unsalted butter

Salt and freshly ground black pepper
2 large eggs
8 ounces Parmesan cheese, grated
Freshly grated nutmeg

Preheat the oven to 350°F. Prepare a 9 × 9-inch casserole dish by rubbing it with the olive oil.

Cut the green stems off the fennel, leaving just the bulb to work with. Trim off the bottom of the bulb. Peel off and discard any damaged outer leaves. Slice the fennel bulb lengthwise into quarters; rinse.

Cut the green tops off the leeks. Trim off the bottom. Slice the leeks in half lengthwise, then cut into pieces about 4 inches long. Rinse well, separating the layers to remove any sand or dirt.

Bring a large pot of salted water to a boil.

Add the leeks and fennel and boil for 15 minutes. Pour the vegetables into a colander to drain. Place the pot back on the stove over medium-high heat. When the pot gets hot, add the butter, then the vegetables, stirring until the fennel and leeks become slightly brown. Season with salt and pepper. Transfer to the casserole dish.

In a bowl, beat the eggs until fluffy. Add 6 ounces of the grated Parmesan to the eggs and stir to combine. Pour the egg mixture over the vegetables. Top with the remaining 2 ounces of cheese and a little nutmeg. Bake for 20 minutes.

Fish and Seafood

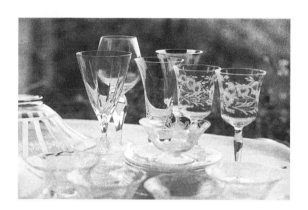

Spicy Rock Shrimp Salad

PROTEINS/FATS AND VEGGIES: LEVEL ONE

SERVES 6

Rock shrimp has a wonderful lobster flavor and combines well with serrano chilies, cilantro, red onions, and lime juice with the added crunch of pickling cucumbers. It's exotic, spicy, and refreshing for a summer salad. Thai fish sauce is available in the Asian foods section of the grocery store or at Asian markets. If you cannot find it, use additional clam juice.

1 pound rock shrimp
1/2 teaspoon salt
1/2 teaspoon white pepper
1/2 cup Thai fish sauce
1 cup fresh lime juice
1/2 cup white vinegar
1/2 cup clam juice

1 medium red onion, finely diced
3 serrano chilies, finely minced, with seeds
2 ripe tomatoes, peeled, seeded, and diced
2 pickling cucumbers, diced with skins on
1 bunch of cilantro
Dash of hot pepper sauce
1 head of green leaf lettuce

Sprinkle the shrimp with the salt and white pepper. Blanch in boiling water for two to three minutes. Drain and chill.

Combine the fish sauce, lime juice, vinegar, clam juice, onion, serranos, tomatoes, cucumbers, and cilantro. Toss well with the chilled rock shrimp. Season with hot pepper sauce and salt and pepper. Using a slot-ted spoon, place a chilled mound of the salad over a green leaf lettuce.

P.S. When working with serrano chilies I always wear kitchen gloves while washing, cutting, and seeding them. When you are finished, thoroughly wash the gloves with hot water and soap. Avoid any direct contact with the eyes while preparing chilies.

Citrus Pesto—Encrusted Fish

PROTEINS/FATS AND VEGGIES: LEVEL ONE

SERVES 2

You won't miss having fish encrusted with bread crumbs when you try this fish rubbed with citrus zest. It's tangy, fresh, and delicious. Try it served over a bed of steamed spinach.

1 small lemon
1 small lime
4 tablespoons olive oil
4 garlic cloves
¼ cup finely chopped parsley
¼ cup finely chopped fresh basil

1 large egg
Salt and freshly ground black pepper
2 fresh sea bass fillets
1 cup dry white wine, reduced
2 tablespoons (¼ stick) unsalted butter

Grate the zest of the lemon and the lime, being careful not to grate the bitter white pith. When finished, squeeze the lemon and lime juice into a bowl and set aside. Place the grated zest, 2 tablespoons of the olive oil, the garlic, parsley, and basil into a food processor. Blend until all the ingredients are finely chopped and well combined. You may need to scrape down the sides. (If you do not have a food processor, chop all the ingredients until very fine and combine.) Pour the mixture onto a plate and set aside.

Place the egg in a shallow bowl and lightly beat. Add salt and pepper. Dip the fish into the egg, then lay the fish on the parsley mixture to coat. Turn over and coat the other side.

Place a skillet over medium-high heat. Add the remaining 2 tablespoons of olive oil, then the fish, and sauté about 4 minutes per side. Remove the fish and set aside to keep warm.

Add the wine to the hot skillet and turn the heat up to high. Let the wine cook off for a couple of minutes, scraping the bits off the bottom of the pan to release the flavors. Add the lemon and lime juice. When the sauce has reduced by half, season with salt and pepper. Turn off the heat and add the butter, 1 tablespoon at a time, swirling until melted.

Serve the fish immediately, with the sauce poured over the top.

Crispy Mesquite Salmon

SERVES 4

I'm very picky when it comes to fish. I buy only the freshest of the fresh. This recipe gives the fish a crispy, herb-crusted shell, while keeping the fish moist and tender. My mother taught me that if you soak fish in milk it removes any fishy smell or flavor. Since milk is a Funky Food, I use cream in this recipe.

1 2-pound fresh salmon or trout fillet, skin
   attached
1 cup light cream
2 tablespoons mayonnaise
Salt and freshly ground black pepper
1 teaspoon dried dill weed

SEASONINGS

1 tablespoon black peppercorns
1 tablespoon green peppercorns
1 teaspoon coriander seeds
1 teaspoon dill seed
2 teaspoons kosher salt

2 lemons, quartered
2 limes, quartered

Preheat the grill to medium-high heat. If you are using a gas grill, buy some mesquite chips and soak them in water for a few hours. Before you light the grill, place the chips around the briquettes.

To prepare the fish, soak the fish in the cream for approximately 30 minutes. Meanwhile, put all the seasonings in a plastic bag and pound them with a mallet to crack the peppercorns and seeds. Remove the fish from the cream. Spread half the mayonnaise on the skin of the fish. Season with salt and pepper. Turn the fish over, exposing the flesh side. Spread the remaining mayonnaise over the flesh and sprinkle with the dried dill weed. Take the seasonings out of the bag and rub them into the flesh. All the flesh should be covered with the mayonnaise and seasonings.

To grill the fish, place the fish on the hot grill, seasoning side down. Cook for 5 to 7 minutes. Turn over with a spatula and grill the other side for an additional 7 minutes, or until the fish flakes when you touch it with a fork. (If you don't have a grill, cook it under the broiler.)

Remove the fish from the grill and place it on a platter, surrounded by lemon and lime wedges.

Herb-Crusted Halibut Steaks with Tomato Basil Sauce

PROTEINS/FATS AND VEGGIES: LEVEL ONE

SERVES 2

This is a light and lovely fish preparation. Try it served over sautéed spinach.

HALIBUT

2 halibut steaks
Salt and freshly ground black pepper
2 tablespoons finely chopped parsley
2 tablespoons finely chopped fresh basil
1 tablespoon olive oil

Rinse the halibut steaks and pat dry. Season both sides of the fish with salt and pepper. Combine the parsley and chopped basil in a small bowl. Make an herb crust on the halibut steaks by pressing the herbs onto both sides of the flesh.

Heat a large skillet over medium-high heat. Add the olive oil, then the fish, and cook for about 3 minutes on each side. Remove the fish and set aside to keep warm.

TOMATO BASIL SAUCE

1 cup dry white wine
1 cup chopped tomatoes
2 tablespoons fresh basil, cut into julienne
1 tablespoon butter

Add the white wine to the hot pan, scraping the bits off the bottom of the pan to release the flavor. When the wine has reduced by about one third, add the tomatoes and basil and stir until just heated through. Turn off the heat and add the butter, swirling until combined.

Serve the halibut steaks with the tomato basil sauce poured over the top.

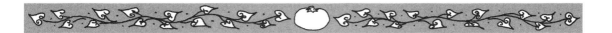

Poultry

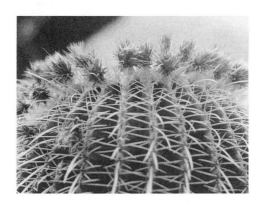

Chinese Chicken Salad

SERVES 4

Most Chinese chicken salads have loads of fried wontons and rice noodles without a lot of flavor. This one's made with marinated chicken and braised green beans. It's perfectly Somersized.

DRESSING

2 tablespoons rice vinegar
Juice of 1/2 lemon
1 tablespoon soy sauce
Freshly ground black pepper
5 tablespoons extra-virgin olive oil
1 tablespoon sesame oil

4 boneless and skinless chicken breasts

MARINADE

1/4 cup soy sauce
1/4 cup sesame oil
1/2 teaspoon hot chile oil
3 garlic cloves, pressed
1 tablespoon grated fresh ginger (or
    1 teaspoon dried)
Juice of 1 lemon

1 tablespoon peanut oil
1 pound mixed field greens
1 recipe Asian Braised String Beans (page
    166)

To make the dressing, place the rice vinegar, lemon juice, soy sauce, and pepper to taste in a mixing cup. Add the olive oil and sesame oil in a steady stream, whisking constantly until the oil is emulsified. Set aside.

To make the chicken, slice the chicken breasts into bite-size pieces. Place in a nonmetallic bowl or a sealable plastic bag with all the marinade ingredients and marinate 2 to 24 hours. The longer you marinate, the more intense the flavors.

Heat a wok over high heat. Add 1 tablespoon peanut oil and the chicken pieces. Cook the chicken pieces for about 3 minutes, until cooked through. Set aside. Prepare the Asian Braised String Beans.

Toss the lettuce with the dressing. Arrange the lettuce on 4 plates. Place the hot chicken pieces on the lettuce. Place the braised string beans on the lettuce. Season with freshly ground pepper and serve.

Turkey Salad in Lettuce Cups

PROTEINS/FATS AND VEGGIES: LEVEL ONE

MAKES 4 TO 6 LETTUCE CUPS

The best part about roasting a turkey on Sunday is having leftovers for the rest of the week. Here's a turkey sandwich served in lettuce cups. Try my Thanksgiving Turkey with Mushroom Sausage Stuffing recipe from Eat Great, Lose Weight, *and add a spoonful of stuffing to your lettuce cup.*

TURKEY SALAD

2 cups cooked turkey meat
3 tablespoons mayonnaise
3 celery stalks, finely chopped
5 green onions, finely chopped
1 cup Mushroom Sausage Stuffing (*EGLW,*
    page 167) (optional)
Salt and freshly ground black pepper

    Place all the ingredients for the turkey salad in a bowl (reserve a few green onions for garnish) and mix until well combined. Adjust the seasonings.
    Place a large dollop of turkey salad in each lettuce leaf. Garnish with the reserved green onions. Fold up and eat like a taco.

LETTUCE CUPS

4 to 6 whole iceberg lettuce leaves

For Level Two
Add a spoonful of cranberry sauce as an additional garnish.

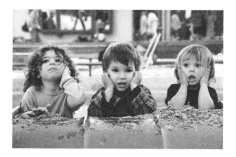

Pretty cute, huh? Three grandchildren.

Grilled Chicken Greek Salad

SERVES 4

I love salads that are hearty enough for an entire meal. This will satisfy your flavor buds and fill your tummy.

4 boneless and skinless chicken breasts
1 cup Lemon Pepper Marinade (page 157)
1 head of romaine lettuce (about 1 pound)
1 large tomato, diced
1/2 red onion, sliced
1 large cucumber, peeled and chopped

1 cup crumbled feta cheese
1 teaspoon dried oregano
1/2 cup extra-virgin olive oil
Juice of 1 lemon
Salt and freshly ground black pepper
8 whole peperoncinis

Preheat the grill to medium heat.

To prepare the chicken, cook the chicken breasts on the hot grill, about 4 minutes per side. (The chicken can be pan-fried if you don't have a grill.) Baste frequently with 1/2 cup of the Lemon Pepper Marinade. (Discard the dressing used to marinate the chicken because it may contain uncooked bacteria from the chicken.) When cooked, place the grilled chicken breasts on a platter and drizzle 1/2 cup more of the Lemon Pep-per Marinade over them. Set aside.

In a salad bowl, toss the lettuce, tomato, onion, cucumber, feta, and oregano with 1/2 cup of olive oil and the lemon juice. Season with salt and pepper. Divide among 4 plates. Slice each chicken breast into 1/2-inch strips and lay on top of each salad. Garnish with the peperoncinis.

For Level Two
Add a handful of kalamata olives.

Chicken Breasts Stuffed with Goat Cheese–Cilantro Pesto

PROTEINS/FATS AND VEGGIES: LEVEL ONE

SERVES 4

Bruce and Caroline made this Southwestern entrée for me at my birthday luncheon. The chicken is grilled, then stuffed under the skin with a creamy goat cheese–cilantro mixture with a kick from serrano chilies. Serve this with Pico de Gallo (page 154) and Tomatillo Salsa (page 154). It's a joy to have children, especially when they can cook!

4 boneless chicken breasts (with skin attached)
¼ cup finely chopped cilantro leaves
¼ cup chicken stock (pages 123 and 125)
2 tablespoons olive oil
Salt and freshly ground black pepper

STUFFING

2 garlic cloves
2 serrano chilies
2 cups cilantro leaves
2 tablespoons olive oil
2 tablespoons freshly grated Parmesan cheese
3 ounces goat cheese
¼ cup ricotta cheese
Salt and freshly ground black pepper

Preheat a grill.

In a nonmetallic container or a sealable plastic bag, place the cilantro leaves, stock, oil, and salt and pepper to taste. Marinate the breasts for 15 minutes, then drain, reserving the marinade.

Place the breasts on the grill, skin side down, and partially cook, 2 to 3 minutes per side, brushing frequently with the marinade. Remove and set aside.

Preheat the oven to 375°F.

In a blender or food processor, puree the garlic, chilies, cilantro, oil, and Parmesan, goat, and ricotta cheeses. Season with salt and pepper. Stuff this mixture under the skin of the chicken breasts, creating an even layer of stuffing. Place in the refrigerator until ready to use. The chicken breasts can be prepared up to this point 6 hours before baking. Make sure to let them sit at room temperature for 15 minutes before baking.

Place the breasts in a roasting pan and pour some of the reserved marinade over them. Bake for 12 minutes and serve immediately.

Chicken Sausage Cassoulet

PROTEINS/FATS AND VEGGIES: LEVEL ONE

SERVES 6

This recipe is best made with homemade chicken broth and leftover chicken. If you don't have leftovers, a large cooked rotisserie chicken from the deli and 4 cans of chicken stock will do. To enrich the flavor of canned broth, simmer the bones of the chicken in the canned broth for about 15 minutes.

2 tablespoons olive oil
1/2 cup chopped sweet onion
1 cup chopped celery
2 garlic cloves, minced
1 large red bell pepper, chopped
2 to 3 chicken sausages, sliced 1/4 inch
    thick
4 cups chicken stock (pages 123 and 125)
1/2 cup dry white wine
1 cup seeded and chopped tomatoes

8 thyme sprigs
1/2 cup chopped parsley
4 cups cooked chicken, shredded
Salt and freshly ground black pepper
3 large okra, sliced (when in season)
1/2 teaspoon cayenne

GARNISH

3 green onions, chopped

Place a large stockpot over medium heat. Add the olive oil and the onions and sauté until the onions are golden brown and caramelized, about 15 minutes. Add the celery and continue cooking over medium heat until the celery is tender. Add the garlic, red pepper, and sausages and cook until the sausages start to brown and the pepper is tender when pierced with a fork. Add the chicken stock and wine. Increase the heat to medium-high and cook for about 10 minutes to reduce a bit and burn off the alcohol.

Add the tomatoes and continue cooking over medium-high heat while the broth continues to reduce. Add the thyme sprigs, parsley, and chicken. Season with salt and pepper and cook over medium heat for about 20 minutes.

Remove the thyme sprigs, then add the okra and cayenne. Continue cooking for another 10 minutes until the okra is soft.

Serve in bowls and garnish with the chopped green onions.

Butterflied Chicken with Zucchini-Ricotta Stuffing

PROTEINS/FATS AND VEGGIES: LEVEL ONE

SERVES 4 TO 6

Stuffing under the skin of the chicken flavors the entire bird. Plus, it's a wonderful way to have stuffing with every bite.

1 6-pound roasting chicken (have your butcher butterfly the chicken by cracking the breastbone so it will lie flat in the roasting pan)
4 large zucchini
Salt
2 tablespoons olive oil, plus extra for rubbing

3 garlic cloves, minced
1 15-ounce carton whole-milk ricotta cheese
Freshly ground black pepper
1 tablespoon herbes de Provence
2 tablespoons (¼ stick) butter

Preheat the oven to 350°F.

To prepare the chicken, clean the chicken thoroughly and pat it dry with paper towels. Lay the chicken flat in the roasting pan. Gently separate the skin of the chicken with your hand, starting at the neck. Put your hand between the skin and the chicken meat and keep separating until the skin is loosened all the way to the bottom of the legs.

To make the stuffing, shred the zucchini by grating it with the large size circular holes of a grater. To help remove some of the excess water found in zucchini, place the shredded zucchini in a colander. Toss with 2 tablespoons of salt and let sit for 20 minutes. During this time, periodically pick up the shredded zucchini with your hands and squeeze it to remove the water. When the zucchini seems to have lost its excess water, rinse to remove the salt. Squeeze the water out one last time.

Place a small skillet over medium heat. Add the olive oil and garlic. Sauté the garlic until golden, about 1 minute. Overcooked garlic will taste bitter.

In a bowl, place the zucchini, sautéed garlic, ricotta, and salt and pepper to taste. Using your hands, mix the ingredients thoroughly.

To stuff the chicken, stuff the zucchini-ricotta mixture *under* the skin of the chicken all the way down to the legs. (When finished, the chicken should look bloated.) Rub the skin with olive oil, salt, pepper, and herbes de Provence. Dot with butter.

Bake for 1½ hours. To carve, cut off leg and thigh pieces whole. Cut off wings. Slice the breast meat into large pieces to keep the stuffing intact.

Shanti's Chicken Curry

SERVES 4

My housekeeper, Shanti, makes a fabulous spicy chicken curry. She was kind enough to share her recipe with me. The main spice is Garam Masala Curry Powder, which is a brown curry. If you can't find that kind, look for another brown curry rather than yellow curry. Serve this with Cucumber Salad (page 136, Proteins/Fats and Veggies version) to cool the spiciness of the dish.

2 tablespoons vegetable oil
1 medium onion, finely chopped
1 tablespoon grated fresh ginger
1 tablespoon minced garlic
4 boneless and skinless chicken breasts, chopped into bite-size pieces
2 tomatoes, finely chopped, with juice and seeds

½ cup cilantro, finely chopped
1 tablespoon Garam Masala Curry Powder
1 tablespoon ground cumin
½ teaspoon chili powder
Salt and freshly ground black pepper

Place the oil in a large skillet over medium-high heat. When hot, add the onion and sauté until translucent, about 4 minutes. Add the ginger and garlic and sauté for 2 minutes longer. Add the chicken and sauté approximately 4 minutes. Add the tomatoes with their juice, the cilantro, curry, cumin, chili powder, and salt and pepper to taste. Stir until the chicken is well coated with the spices.

Cover, lower the heat, and simmer for about 30 minutes. As it cooks, the juice from the tomatoes will absorb into the chicken. (If there is not enough liquid, you should add a little water.) After 30 minutes, if there is still liquid left in the pan, uncover it, turn up the heat to medium, and cook off the liquid. Serve with Cucumber Salad.

Farm-Raised Chicken St. Germain Beaupré

PROTEINS/FATS AND VEGGIES: LEVEL ONE

SERVES 4 TO 6

This is an unusual and delicious way to prepare a chicken that my dear friend Mizou (my stepson Stephen's mother-in-law) taught me. Parboiling the chicken first removes a lot of the fat and allows for a shorter roasting time, which leaves the chicken very moist and juicy with crispy, crackling skin. You must try this! I serve it with Mushroom-Shallot Dressing (page 165).

Salt
1 5- to 7-pound chicken (organic, farm-raised, if possible)
3 tablespoons olive oil
Freshly ground black pepper
4 to 6 fresh tarragon sprigs (or 2 tablespoons dried)
1 tablespoon herbes de Provence

3 tablespoons butter
3 whole onions, quartered

PAN DRIPPINGS

2 cups boiling chicken water
2 tablespoons (¼ stick) unsalted butter
Salt and freshly ground black pepper

Preheat the oven to 350° F.

Fill your largest stockpot halfway with water and add 1 teaspoon of salt. Bring to a boil. Add the chicken and cover. Continue boiling on the stovetop for 20 to 25 minutes. Carefully lift out the chicken and reserve 2 cups of the water.

Place the parboiled chicken in a large roasting pan. Brush the outside of the chicken with olive oil, salt, pepper, fresh tarragon (place 1 tarragon sprig inside the cavity), and herbes de Provence. Dot the chicken all over with pats of butter. Rub the quartered onions with olive oil and place around the chicken in the roasting pan.

Place the pan in the hot oven for 35 to 40 minutes, basting often with pan juices. The bird is done when the skin is crispy brown and crackling and the leg jiggles back and forth easily. Remove from the oven and reserve the pan juices. Place the chicken on a platter. Leave the onions in the roasting pan. You do not have to pour the fat off from the pan because most of the fat was removed during the boiling process. Put the roasting pan on the stove over high heat. Pour in the 2 cups reserved boiling chicken water and bring to a boil. Scrape the bits off the bottom of the pan to release the flavor. Reduce the sauce by one half. Turn off the heat. Add the butter, 1 tablespoon at a time, swirling until melted. Add salt and pepper to taste. Serve the sauce over the carved bird.

Crunchy Roasted Lemon Chicken

PROTEINS/FATS AND VEGGIES: LEVEL ONE

SERVES 4

I love crispy, crunchy skin on my chicken. This technique does the trick.

4 chicken legs
4 chicken breasts, halved widthwise

MARINADE

2 cups fresh lemon juice
1 cup extra-virgin olive oil
1 tablespoon balsamic vinegar
2 blanched garlic cloves (see Note)

1 teaspoon dried oregano
Salt and freshly ground black pepper

SAUCE

1 cup chicken stock (pages 123 and 125)

GARNISH

1 bunch of parsley

Combine the chicken and marinade ingredients in a nonmetallic bowl. Cover with plastic wrap and marinate the chicken for at least 15 minutes. (The flavor is great if it marinates for up to 24 hours in the refrigerator.)

Place the top rack in the oven at least 6 inches from the broiler. Preheat the broiler. Remove the chicken pieces from the marinade and place them in a roasting pan, skin side down for the breasts. Reserve the marinade. Broil the chicken for 15 minutes. Remove the pan from the broiler and using tongs, dip each chicken piece back into the marinade. Place the chicken back into the roasting pan, skin side up, and broil for 10 more minutes. Again, remove the pan from the oven and dip the chicken pieces back into the marinade, then broil for 2 to 3 more minutes.

Remove the chicken from the pan and place on a platter. Place the hot roasting pan on the stove over medium-high heat. Scrape the bits off the bottom of the pan for about 3 minutes. Add the chicken stock and continue scraping the bits until the sauce reduces by half. Pour the sauce over the chicken and garnish with the parsley.

Note
To blanch garlic, place water in a saucepan and bring to a boil. Put one whole unpeeled head of garlic into the boiling water. When the water returns to a boil, remove the garlic and submerge in cold water. Peel the garlic and put it back into the boiling water for a minute. Drain the water and store the garlic until ready to use.

Balsamic Roast Chicken

PROTEINS/FATS AND VEGGIES: LEVEL ONE

SERVES 4 TO 6

Balsamic vinegar is aged in wooden casks, giving it a strong, sweet flavor. Wait'll you taste what it does for this chicken! It's excellent served with Grilled Radicchio (page 177).

1 5- to 6-pound whole chicken (organic, hormone-free is best)
2 tablespoons chopped fresh rosemary
2 tablespoons sea salt
3 garlic cloves, chopped
1 tablespoon freshly ground black pepper
2 red onions, chopped
1/4 cup balsamic vinegar
1/4 cup good red table wine (the better the wine, the better the flavor)

Preheat the oven to 350°F.

To clean the chicken, remove any fatty pieces. Pull out the neck, giblets, and liver and reserve. Rinse the bird and pat it dry.

In a small dish, combine the rosemary, sea salt, garlic, and pepper. Rub this mixture all over the raw chicken inside and out. Let sit for at least 1 hour. You can do this step up to 24 hours in advance so the flavors take hold. Cover the chicken and place in the refrigerator.

Place the neck, giblets, and liver on the bottom of a roasting pan. Sprinkle the chopped red onions on top. Then place the whole chicken on top of the onions. Pour the balsamic vinegar and wine over the chicken.

Roast the chicken in the oven for approximately 2 hours (20 minutes per pound).

Carve the chicken and serve with the balsamic and onion mixture from the bottom of the pan.

Grilled Chicken with Tuscan Artichoke Pâté

PROTEINS/FATS AND VEGGIES: LEVEL ONE

SERVES 4

Tuscan Artichoke Pâté works perfectly with grilled chicken. Garnish with thin lemon slices for a lovely presentation.

4 boneless and skinless chicken breast
   halves
½ cup fresh lemon juice
½ cup extra-virgin olive oil
1 tablespoon lemon zest
1 teaspoon black peppercorns, cracked
1 recipe Tuscan Artichoke Pâté (page 174)
1 teaspoon chopped fresh thyme

GARNISH

1 lemon, thinly sliced
1 teaspoon chopped fresh thyme leaves

To make the chicken, place the chicken breasts in a nonmetallic bowl or plastic freezer bag with half of the fresh lemon juice, the olive oil, lemon zest, cracked peppercorns, and thyme leaves. Marinate for at least 30 minutes or up to 3 hours.

Preheat the grill to medium-high heat. (The chicken breasts can be broiled if you do not have a grill.) When the grill is hot, place the chicken on it. Grill the breasts 4 to 6 minutes on each side, basting frequently with the marinade.

Place some artichoke pâté on each plate. Place a chicken breast on top of the pâté and garnish with thin slices of lemon and a sprinkle of fresh thyme.

Chicken Scaloppine with Tarragon

PROTEINS/FATS AND VEGGIES: LEVEL ONE

SERVES 4

One can never have enough good chicken recipes. This is a variation of Turkey Prosciutto Piccata with Port Glaze (page 200).

8 chicken cutlets (breast slices pounded to paper-thin scaloppine—your butcher will do this for you if you ask)
Salt and freshly ground black pepper
8 fresh tarragon sprigs
8 paper-thin slices of pancetta (prosciutto or regular bacon can be substituted)

2 tablespoons olive oil
3 tablespoons butter
1/2 cup dry white wine
1/2 cup chicken stock (pages 123 and 125)
4 lemon wedges

To prepare the cutlets, season both sides of the cutlets with salt and pepper. Place 1 large tarragon sprig on each piece of turkey. On top of the cutlet and tarragon, place 1 piece of pancetta. Press the tarragon and pancetta against the cutlet to make them stick. Repeat until all the cutlets are prepared.

(The cutlets may be prepared as above up to 4 hours in advance. Cover them and place in the refrigerator. Just make sure you remove them from the refrigerator 15 minutes before cooking to allow them to come to room temperature. Otherwise they will be tough.)

To cook the cutlets, place a large skillet over medium-high heat. Add the olive oil and 2 tablespoons of butter. When the butter is melted, add as many cutlets as will fit flat in the pan. Cook for 2 minutes on each side. As the cutlets are cooked, set aside in a warm oven. Continue until all the cutlets are cooked.

To make the sauce, after removing the last cutlets from the frying pan, add the wine. Cook until the steam disappears. Add the chicken stock, then reduce the sauce by half, turn off the heat, and stir in the remaining 1 tablespoon of butter until melted.

Place 2 cutlets on each plate and top with a little sauce. Serve with a lemon wedge.

Turkey Prosciutto Piccata with Port Glaze

SERVES 6

This is an incredible recipe from my good friend Wolfgang Puck. He has taught me so much about cooking! I am constantly inspired by his talent. This is great served with Celery Root Puree with Crispy Fried Onions (page 169). The turkey cutlets used in this recipe are made from slices of turkey breast that are pounded until they are paper thin. Ask your butcher to prepare them for you.

12 turkey cutlets (breast slices, flattened until paper thin)
Salt and freshly ground black pepper
24 fresh sage leaves (if not available, use 2 tablespoons powdered sage)
12 paper-thin slices of prosciutto (a salty Italian ham usually available at an Italian deli)

3 tablespoons olive oil
3 tablespoons butter
$\frac{1}{2}$ cup port wine

To prepare the cutlets, season both sides of the cutlets with salt and pepper. Place 2 sage leaves onto each piece of turkey. On top of the cutlet and sage place 1 piece of prosciutto. Press the sage and prosciutto against the cutlet to make them stick. Repeat until all the cutlets are prepared. (The cutlets may be prepared to this point up to 4 hours in advance. Cover them and place in the refrigerator. Just make sure you remove them from the refrigerator 15 minutes before cooking to let the meat come to room temperature. Otherwise they will be tough.)

To cook the cutlets, put the olive oil and 2 tablespoons of butter in a large frying pan. When the butter is melted, add as many cutlets as will fit flat in the pan. Cook for 2 minutes on each side. As the cutlets are cooked, set them aside in a warm oven. Continue until all the cutlets are cooked.

To make the sauce, after removing the last cutlets from the frying pan, add the port wine. Cook until the steam disappears. Reduce the sauce by half, then turn off the heat and stir in the remaining 1 tablespoon butter until melted.

Place 2 cutlets on each plate and top with a little sauce.

Roast Christmas Goose with Port Glaze

SERVES 4 TO 6

Everyone seems to be afraid of cooking a goose. Trust me, it's easy. You usually have to order a goose in advance from your butcher. Request a large one—10 to 14 pounds. There is a lot of shrinkage. One goose serves 4 to 6 people. Order two if you are giving a larger dinner.

1 10- to 14-pound goose
1 onion, halved
2 teaspoons chopped fresh thyme
Salt and freshly ground black pepper
3 tablespoons olive oil
1 tablespoon dried sage
1 tablespoon dried thyme
1 tablespoon poultry seasoning
1 tablespoon allspice

PORT SAUCE

Goose giblets (except the liver)
4 celery stalks
3 garlic cloves, peeled
1 large onion, chopped
4 parsley sprigs
1 cup port wine
1 box dried currants, soaked in water until
    soft
Salt and freshly ground black pepper

Preheat the oven to 350°F.

Clean the goose thoroughly and remove any extra fatty pieces. Reserve the giblets for the sauce. Stuff the goose with 2 onion halves, fresh thyme, and salt and pepper to taste.

Rub the goose with olive oil. Season with about 1 tablespoon each of the following: salt, pepper, dried sage, dried thyme, poultry seasoning, and allspice. Prick the bird all over with a fork lightly to allow the excess fat to escape.

Roast the goose on a rack in a roasting pan for 20 to 25 minutes per pound, basting occasionally. The bird is done when the legs jiggle easily and the juices run clear when the skin is pierced.

While the goose is roasting, place the giblets, celery, garlic, onion, parsley, and 6 cups of water in a saucepan and bring to a boil. Reduce the heat and skim the foam off the top. Simmer for 2 hours. Strain, reserving the stock. Finely chop the giblets and set aside. Remove the goose from the pan and skim almost all the fat from the juices with a large spoon. Place the roasting pan with goose drippings over medium heat. Scrape the particles on the bottom of the pan. Add the port, 2 cups of stock, and the chopped giblets. Reduce over high heat, stirring for about 15 minutes, or until slightly thickened. Add the drained currants. Add salt and pepper to taste.

Pour the port sauce over the carved goose.

Pierre's New Year's Eve Stuffed Roast Capon

PROTEINS/FATS AND VEGGIES: LEVEL ONE

SERVES 8 TO 10

My friend Pierre shared this fabulous recipe with me. It is different because the stuffing is placed under the skin of the bird. I make it once a year because it's expensive but worth it. Capons are roosters with exceptionally tender flesh. If your butcher cannot order one for you, an organic chicken or turkey will do. The fois gras and truffles can be ordered in advance from the Dean & Deluca food catalog, 1-800-221-7714. (Ask for prices first.) This recipe is failproof and unbelievably good. The stuffing is very rich, so you won't miss potatoes or other filler foods. I like to start this meal with Endive and Radicchio Salad with Stilton Cheese (page 141) and then serve the capon with buttered haricots verts (baby string beans) tied in bundles. Have fun and Happy New Year!

1 8-pound organic capon (or chicken or turkey)

Salt

1 pound ground veal (if you don't eat veal, ground turkey will do)

1 pound ground pork

6 to 8 ounces fois gras (or, if unavailable, 6 to 8 ounces fresh chicken livers sautéed in butter until cooked through, 8 to 10 minutes on medium heat. When cool, finely chop the livers in a food processor.)

1 cup favorite Cognac or bourbon

1 whole black truffle, optional (very expensive but delicious)

2 tablespoons olive oil

6 tablespoons butter

Freshly ground black pepper

1 whole onion

2 celery stalks, cut in half

1 cup Rich Capon Stock (page 122)

PAN DRIPPINGS

2 cups capon stock (page 122)

4 tablespoons (½ stick) unsalted butter

Preheat the oven to 350°F.

Clean the capon and rub inside and out with salt. Remove the giblets and neck and reserve for the stock. The stuffing for the capon will go between the skin and the meat. Begin by loosening the skin at the neck with your hands. Gently loosen the skin from the meat all the way to the legs and thighs. Set aside.

For the stuffing, in a large bowl, place the veal, pork, fois gras, and Cognac or bourbon. Knead together with your hands until well blended. Gently cut off the rough outer shell of the truffle, if using, with a small sharp knife. Then cut the truffle into paper-thin slices and add to the stuffing mixture. Using your hands, push the stuffing mixture under the skin of the capon, making sure you fill every inch of space (legs, thighs, and breast).

Rub the outside of the capon with olive oil and butter. Sprinkle with salt and pepper. Place the onion and celery stalks in the cavity of the bird. Place the stuffed bird in a large roasting pan.

Pour 1 cup of capon stock into the bottom of the roasting pan. Place the roasting pan in the preheated oven. Cook for 3 hours 20 minutes (25 minutes per pound). Baste occasionally during the cooking time with the pan juices. You can tell the doneness if the leg moves easily when jiggled.

When the bird is done, remove from the roasting pan. Pour off most of the fat from the roasting pan, leaving about $1/4$ cup. Put the roasting pan on the stovetop over medium-high heat. When the pan gets hot, add 2 cups of capon stock and let cook until the liquid is reduced by half. Scrape the bits off the bottom of the pan to release the flavor. Add salt to taste.

Turn off the heat and add the butter, 1 tablespoon at a time, swirling until melted. Pour into a gravy boat and serve immediately.

Serve each person the capon slices topped with delicious fois gras stuffing and pan drippings.

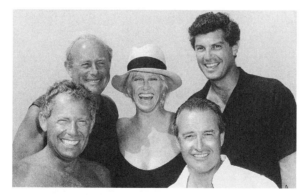

Just the way I like it . . . me and a bunch of handsome guys having fun at the beach in St. Tropez.
Top Row: George, me, and Carl
Bottom Row: My husband Alan and Pierre
(of Pierre's famous New Year's Eve
Stuffed Roast Capon)

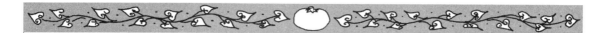

Meat

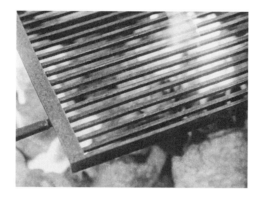

Beef Stroganoff

SERVES 6

In the late sixties beef stroganoff was "the dish" to serve for company. Today it's still a hit, but I don't serve it with fettuccine anymore. Instead I serve it with sautéed spinach. Now when Alan and I eat it, we wear our bell bottoms.

2½ pounds beef tenderloin
1 tablespoon unsalted butter
2½ cups sliced mushrooms
¼ teaspoon salt
Freshly ground black pepper
1½ cups dill pickles, cut into julienne,
    with 2 tablespoons pickle juice

2 cups heavy cream
2 tablespoons vegetable oil
1 recipe Sautéed Spinach with Garlic and
    Olive Oil (page 171)

Trim any silver skin on the tenderloin, then cut across the width into 1-inch slices. Slightly flatten the slices by pressing with the palm of your hand. Set aside.

Place a skillet over medium-high heat, add the butter, and melt. Sauté the mushrooms with salt and pepper until golden, about 5 minutes. Add the pickles and juice, and cook until the juice evaporates slightly, about 2 minutes. Add the cream and cook until reduced by half.

Meanwhile, season the meat with a little salt and pepper (the sauce will be salty from the pickles). Heat a large skillet over high heat, add the oil, and heat until it starts smoking. Sear the meat briefly, 2 minutes per side for medium rare. Place the sautéed spinach on the plates, top with the beef, then ladle the warm sauce over the top.

P.S. I know the dill pickle sounds weird, but try it—you will love it.

Filets Mignons au Poivre

SERVES 4

There's nothing like a little beef and filet mignon is the perfect little beef.

4 6-ounce bacon-wrapped filets mignons
Salt
1 tablespoon white peppercorns
1 tablespoon black peppercorns
2 tablespoons (¼ stick) unsalted butter

1 tablespoon olive oil
2 tablespoons port wine
2 tablespoons beef stock (page 124)
¼ cup heavy cream (optional)

Have your butcher wrap 4 trimmed 6-ounce filets with bacon. Pat the steaks dry with a paper towel and sprinkle with salt. Bring to room temperature.

Place the white and black peppercorns in a small plastic bag and crack with a mallet or the bottom of a pan. Rub the steaks on both sides with salt and the cracked pepper, pushing the peppercorns into the meat.

In a large skillet, heat 1 tablespoon of the butter and the olive oil over medium-high heat. Place the steaks in the pan and cook for 3 to 4 minutes per side for medium rare. Remove the steaks to a platter. Remove the bacon and discard.

Pour off any excess fat from the skillet and return to the heat. Add the port wine and let come to a boil while scraping the bits from the bottom of the pan. Add the beef stock and continue cooking over medium-high heat, reducing the sauce until it is rich and syrupy. Lower the heat and blend in the cream, if desired. Remove from the heat and add the other tablespoon of butter to the sauce and let it melt.

Milanese Beef with Sautéed Onions and Mushrooms in a Port Wine Sauce

PROTEINS/FATS AND VEGGIES: LEVEL ONE

SERVES 4

This is the magnificent meal Caroline and Bruce made for us just before Violet was born. I can still remember Caroline, with her big belly, deglazing the pan with my granddaughter Camelia balanced on her hip. This meal requires a whole bottle of port. Don't forget to try this beef marinade for any of your favorite cuts—it's divine.

MARINADE

½ cup port wine
1 cup olive oil
2 garlic cloves, minced
2 tablespoons dry mustard
2 teaspoons soy sauce
1 teaspoon fresh lemon juice
Salt and freshly ground black pepper
Dash of hot pepper sauce
Dash of Worcestershire sauce (see Note, page 131)

4 Milanese beef cutlets (thinly pounded slices of sirloin steak)

MUSHROOMS AND ONIONS

6 tablespoons olive oil
3 large onions, sliced
1 pound mushrooms
2 teaspoons dried thyme
1 cup beef stock (page 124)
½ cup port wine
Salt and freshly ground black pepper
2 tablespoons (¼ stick) unsalted butter

SAUCE

2 cups port wine
2 tablespoons (¼ stick) unsalted butter

Combine the marinade ingredients in a nonmetallic bowl or a large sealable plastic bag. Add the steaks and marinate 6 to 24 hours, turning the steaks after half the time has passed.

For the mushrooms and onions, heat a large skillet over medium heat. Add 3 tablespoons of olive oil. Add the onions and sauté until they become golden brown and begin to caramelize, about 10 minutes. Add the mushrooms. Continue stirring and add the remaining 3 tablespoons of oil and the dried thyme. As they cook, the mushrooms will release all of their liquid. Continue cooking them down until the liquid has cooked off, approximately 15 minutes. At this point they will begin to get brown and crusty on the edges.

Turn the heat up to high and add ½ cup of port and the beef stock. It should steam immediately. Stir the mushrooms and wine, scraping the bottom of the pan to release the flavor. Add salt and pepper to taste. Continue to cook over high heat until the liquid is reduced by half. Turn off the heat and add the butter. Stir to combine.

To cook the steaks, heat a large skillet over medium-high heat. Remove the steaks from the marinade and place as many as will fit flat in the pan. Cook for 2 minutes on each side. Remove and set aside in a warm place until all the steaks are cooked. When all are cooked, place the pan over high heat and add 2 cups of port. Scrape the bits off the bottom of the pan to release the flavor. When the sauce has reduced by half, turn off the heat and add the butter, 1 tablespoon at a time, swirling until combined.

Serve each steak topped with a pile of mushrooms and the port sauce.

Persian Kabobs

PROTEINS/FATS AND VEGGIES: LEVEL ONE

SERVES 4 TO 6

These kabobs aren't pieces of meat on skewers, they're simply the best hamburgers you've ever eaten! The secret is the grated onion and the Persian seasoning called "Koubideh." Look for it in ethnic markets. If you can't find it, use garlic powder, onion powder, turmeric, and sumac. Serve this with Cucumber Salad (page 136, Proteins/Fats and Veggies version) and Grilled Vegetable Tower (page 168).

1 grated onion, with juice
2 pounds ground beef

2 tablespoons "Koubideh" Persian kabob
   seasoning

Grate the onion over a plate to catch all the juices. Combine the hamburger meat with the grated onion and juices. Add the Koubideh and mash together with your hands until well combined. Refrigerate 6 to 24 hours. The longer the meat sits, the better the flavor.

Preheat the grill to medium-high heat.

Form the meat into ¼-pound egg-shaped patties. You don't want them completely flattened but slightly dome shaped.

Grill over medium-high heat for 8 to 10 minutes, turning frequently to brown all sides.

Grilled Steaks Provençal

SERVES 4

We especially love this simple steak meal in the summer. The peppers add an incredible flavor and look simply beautiful. And the steak has a clean, fresh taste with just a squeeze of lemon. Yum.

4 porterhouse steaks, approximately 8
   ounces each
8 tablespoons olive oil
Salt and coarsely ground black pepper
2 medium sweet onions (Vidalia or Maui),
   cut into julienne

2 medium red bell peppers, cut into
   julienne
2 medium yellow bell peppers, cut into
   julienne
1 tablespoon butter
1 lemon, quartered

Preheat the grill to medium-high heat.

To prepare the steaks, trim the excess fat from the steaks and let sit at room temperature for 10 minutes. Rub the steaks on both sides with 4 tablespoons of olive oil and salt and pepper to taste.

To prepare the peppers and onions, place a skillet with the remaining 4 tablespoons of olive oil over medium-high heat. Add the onions and peppers and cook until golden brown, approximately 20 to 30 minutes.

Season with salt and pepper. Add the butter and toss well.

To cook the steaks, place the steaks on the hot grill. Cook for 7 minutes per side for medium.

To serve, place a pile of peppers and onions on each plate. Remove the steaks from the grill and place on top of the peppers and onions. Garnish each plate with a lemon wedge to squeeze over the steaks.

Beef Tournedos in Burgundy Sauce

PROTEINS/FATS AND VEGGIES: LEVEL ONE

SERVES 4

These slices of beef are rubbed with baked garlic and finished with a burgundy wine sauce—great flavors!

BAKED GARLIC

1 head of garlic
Olive oil
Fresh or dried thyme

TOURNEDOS

1 pound beef tenderloin, sliced ½ inch thick (ask your butcher to do this for you)

Salt and freshly ground black pepper
2 tablespoons olive oil
1 whole shallot, minced
1 cup beef stock (page 124)
¼ cup burgundy wine
2 tablespoons tomato puree
2 tablespoons (¼ stick) unsalted butter
Chopped parsley

For the baked garlic, preheat the oven to 350°F. Slice the top off the head of garlic, exposing the cluster of cloves. Brush with a touch of olive oil and sprinkle with thyme. Place in a shallow baking dish and bake for 45 minutes, or until golden brown and bubbly. Remove from the heat and set aside.

For the tournedos, squeeze about 8 garlic cloves out of their skins. Rub the filets all over with the roasted garlic cloves. Season with salt and pepper. Heat a skillet over medium-high heat. Add the olive oil and as many of the filets as will fit into the pan. Brown for 2 to 3 minutes per side. Remove from the pan and keep warm. Repeat until all the filets are browned, adding more oil as necessary.

When all the meat is cooked, add the shallot and cook until tender, about 3 minutes. Add the stock and wine. Turn the heat up to high, scraping the bits from the bottom of the pan to release the flavor. Let the sauce reduce by half. Add the tomato puree, stirring until heated through. Turn off the heat and add the butter, 1 tablespoon at a time, until well combined.

Place the filets on a plate and top with the sauce. Garnish with the parsley.

Swedish Meatballs

PROTEINS/FATS AND VEGGIES: LEVEL ONE

SERVES 4

This recipe seems sinful, but it is Level One. The sauce is so rich you don't miss rice or potatoes.

1 pound ground extra-lean beef
1 pound ground pork
1 large egg
2 tablespoons olive oil
1 cup minced onion
½ cup minced celery
3 cups beef stock (page 124)

2 beef bouillon cubes
1 garlic clove
1 teaspoon allspice
Salt and freshly ground black pepper
5 black peppercorns
8 ounces cream cheese
Parsley

Crumble the ground beef and ground pork into a large bowl and add the egg. Set aside.

Place a large skillet over medium-high heat. Add the olive oil and onions. Sauté the onions until translucent, about 5 minutes. Add the celery and cook for 4 minutes more.

While the celery and onions cook, put the stock, bouillon cubes, and garlic into a stockpot and bring to a boil.

Add the onion mixture, allspice, and salt and pepper to taste to the meat. Work the mixture well with your hands, blending all the flavors together. Form the meat into tiny 1-inch balls and place them on a cookie sheet lined with wax paper. You should have 30 to 40 meatballs.

Slowly add the meatballs, one at a time, to the boiling stock. Depending upon the size of the stockpot you use, you may have to cook the meatballs in 2 batches. Add the peppercorns at this time. Let the meatballs cook for about 20 minutes.

Remove the meatballs from the stock with a slotted spoon and set aside. Strain the stock. Place the stock back in the pot over medium-high heat. Reduce the stock for about 10 minutes. Turn off the heat and add the cream cheese, whisking until well combined. Pour the rich, creamy beef sauce over the meatballs and garnish with parsley.

Pan-Fried New York Steak with Fried Elephant Garlic

PROTEINS/FATS AND VEGGIES: LEVEL ONE

SERVES 2

I first tasted steak cooked this way when Alan and I were traveling in Tuscany. It takes 15 minutes to prepare, which is the best news of all. The steaks are cooked in olive oil infused with hot chilies, rosemary, and elephant garlic. If you don't have elephant garlic, regular garlic works great. I love this meal with a big salad and sautéed spinach.

2 tablespoons black peppercorns
2¼-inch-thick New York steaks (ask your
    butcher to pound them for you)
⅓ cup extra-virgin olive oil
4 elephant garlic cloves (or 8 regular
    cloves), thinly sliced

2 teaspoons salt
1 tablespoon rosemary leaves
4 fresh rosemary sprigs (or 4 teaspoons
    dried)
4 whole dried red chile peppers

Place the peppercorns in a plastic bag and crack them with the bottom of a pan or a mallet. Brush the steaks with a little olive oil. Rub one of the sliced garlic cloves over both sides of the meat. Combine the salt, freshly cracked peppercorns, and 1 tablespoon rosemary leaves. Use this mixture to season the steaks on both sides.

Heat a skillet with the olive oil over medium heat. When it's hot, add the rest of the sliced garlic and sauté until golden brown, about 5 minutes. Remove the garlic

and set aside. Add the rosemary sprigs, pressing them flat against the bottom of the skillet with a spatula to get them crispy, about 2 minutes on each side. Remove and set aside. Add the chilies and toss in the hot oil for 30 seconds. Remove and set aside.

Fry the steaks in the infused hot oil, adding more oil if necessary, 2 to 3 minutes on each side.

Top the steaks with the garlic, rosemary sprigs, and chilies. Serve immediately.

Rosemary London Broil

SERVES 4

There's nothing like a great steak. For many years, when I still bought into the low-fat movement, I stayed away from meat and ate mostly chicken. Boy, did I get tired of chicken! Now I enjoy beef frequently. Here's a delicious way to prepare London broil. This meal is great with some grilled mushrooms and a salad with Roquefort Dressing (EGLW, page 108).

1 teaspoon black peppercorns
2 garlic cloves, pressed
2 tablespoons chopped fresh rosemary
1 tablespoon grated lemon zest

2 tablespoons olive oil
1 cup dry red wine
1 2-pound London broil
2 tablespoons (¼ stick) butter

Place the peppercorns in a plastic bag and seal. Pound with a mallet or the bottom of a frying pan to crack the peppercorns.

In a large nonmetallic bowl or sealable plastic bag, place the garlic and rosemary. With a large spoon, mash or press the garlic and rosemary, releasing the flavors. Add the cracked peppercorns and lemon zest and mash together. Add the oil and half the red wine.

Remove the meat from the refrigerator and score on the top and bottom with a knife by cutting an **X** into the meat about ⅛ inch thick. Place the meat in the marinade for at least 15 minutes, turning after half the time has expired. The flavor is best if it's marinated overnight.

Preheat the grill to high heat. Remove the meat from the marinade and place it on the grill. For medium rare, the meat will take approximately 5 minutes per side for a 1½-inch-thick London broil.

Meanwhile, strain the marinade. Discard the rosemary, peppercorns, and lemon zest. Place the liquid in a skillet over high heat. Let the marinade reduce by about one third. Add the remaining red wine. Let the liquid reduce by half, then turn off the heat. Add the butter, 1 tablespoon at a time, and stir until melted.

When the meat is cooked, let it rest for 10 minutes. Thinly slice it on an angle and serve with the sauce.

Picadillo

SERVES 8

Rita Moreno taught me how to make this on my talk show and I absolutely loved it! Picadillo is a Puerto Rican staple. Some wonderful Puerto Rican housewife probably discovered this by adding everything but the kitchen sink.

2 tablespoons olive oil
2 medium onions, finely chopped
1 large bell pepper, finely chopped
6 plum tomatoes, chopped
Salt and freshly ground black pepper
1 teaspoon minced fresh garlic
1 teaspoon ground cumin
1 teaspoon ground coriander
1 pound lean ground beef

1 pound pork
¾ cup balsamic vinegar
2 tablespoons capers, drained
½ cup tomato puree

GARNISH

Sour cream
1 bunch of cilantro, chopped
1 head of iceberg lettuce

Heat the olive oil in a large skillet over medium heat. Add the onions and peppers. Cook until they are brown and tender, 10 to 15 minutes. Then add the tomatoes, salt and pepper to taste, garlic, cumin, and coriander.

Turn the heat up to medium-high and add the meat. Brown the meat, using a wooden spoon to break it into tiny pieces.

Add the balsamic vinegar, capers, and tomato puree. Reduce the heat and simmer for at least 1 hour.

Serve in a bowl with a dollop of sour cream and chopped cilantro. Or roll up in a lettuce leaf and eat like a taco.

For Level Two
Add ¼ cup chopped black olives.

Lamb Shanks with Oregano and Feta

PROTEINS/FATS AND VEGGIES: LEVEL ONE

SERVES 4

I love peasant dishes. These lamb shanks are an inexpensive way to serve lamb, and they're loaded with flavor. They slow cook until the meat falls off the bone. This is Alan's favorite dinner. He oohs and ahhs; has seconds and sometimes thirds.

4 lamb shanks
Salt and freshly ground black pepper
1/2 cup olive oil
3 medium onions, thinly sliced
6 cups chicken stock (pages 123 and 125)

3 tablespoons chopped fresh oregano leaves
   or 2 tablespoons dried
1/4 teaspoon cayenne
1 28-ounce can peeled tomatoes, chopped,
   with juice
1 cup crumbled feta cheese

Trim any excess fat from the shanks, then season with salt and pepper. Heat the oil in a stockpot over high heat. Add the shanks, turning frequently to brown all sides. Remove from the pot and reserve.

Lower the heat to medium and add the onions, stirring until golden brown, about 7 to 10 minutes. Add the stock, oregano leaves, cayenne, and tomatoes with juice. Scrape the bits off the bottom of the pan to release the flavor. Add the shanks back to the pan. (If the shanks are not completely covered by liquid, add enough water to cover.) Bring to a boil, then lower the heat and simmer for about 2 1/2 hours. The shanks are done when the meat is practically falling off the bone.

To serve, arrange 1 shank per person in your favorite bowls. Sprinkle with feta cheese and top with the onions and the sauce. Serve immediately.

For Level Two
Serve the shanks over a bowl of whole-wheat couscous, available in health food and Middle Eastern stores.

Roasted Leg of Lamb

PROTEINS/FATS AND VEGGIES: LEVEL ONE

SERVES 8 TO 10

Nothing makes the house smell better than a leg of lamb roasting in the oven. I like to cover mine with loads of fresh garlic inserted into the flesh.

1 7- to 8-pound whole leg of lamb
8 garlic cloves, halved
2 tablespoons olive oil
2 tablespoons dried rosemary
2 tablespoons dried thyme
Salt and freshly ground black pepper

PAN DRIPPINGS

1 cup lamb or beef stock (page 124)
1 cup red wine
2 tablespoons butter

Preheat the oven to 350°F.

Using a small paring knife, make 16 small slits into the flesh of the lamb. Insert half a clove of garlic into each slit. Rub the lamb with the olive oil, then sprinkle with the rosemary, thyme, and salt and plenty of freshly ground pepper.

Place the lamb, fat side up, on a rack in a roasting pan. Set the pan in the oven and roast for 1¼ to 1½ hours. Baste several times during cooking with the accumulated juices. After 1 hour, start testing for doneness with a meat thermometer: 130°F. for medium rare, 140°F. for medium.

As soon as the lamb is done, remove it from the roasting pan and set aside for carving. Pour off most of the fat from the roasting pan, reserving about 3 tablespoons to make the sauce. Place the roasting pan on top of the stove over high heat. When the pan is good and hot, add the stock and wine, scraping the bits from the bottom of the pan to release the flavors. Let the sauce reduce by one half. Turn off the heat and add the butter, 1 tablespoon at a time, swirling until melted and combined. Spoon the sauce over the carved meat.

Lamb Skewers with Harissa Dipping Sauce

PROTEINS/FATS AND VEGGIES: LEVEL ONE

MAKES 25 TO 30 SKEWERS AND 1½ CUPS SAUCE

Ken Brown's delicious creation with a spicy Mediterranean sauce was the perfect passed hors d'oeuvre at my granddaughter's christening. Have your butcher give you a rack of lamb, minus the bones.

LAMB SKEWERS

3 pounds lamb loin
2 tablespoons ground cumin
2 tablespoons ground coriander
2 teaspoons kosher slat
⅓ cup olive oil
3 tablespoons minced garlic

Preheat the grill to high heat.

Cut the lamb into 1- to 2-inch bite-size strips. Toss with the remaining ingredients and marinate for 3 to 4 hours or overnight. Place the lamb on skewers (1 piece per skewer), then grill or broil for 2 to 3 minutes, turning frequently.

HARISSA SAUCE

2 red bell peppers, roasted and peeled
1 tablespoon ground cumin
1 teaspoon sweet paprika
2 teaspoons kosher salt
2 tablespoons extra-virgin olive oil
1 teaspoon fresh lemon juice

For the harissa sauce, combine all the ingredients in a blender and blend until smooth. Serve at room temperature with the lamb skewers.

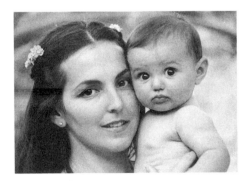

Caroline and our beautiful new granddaughter Violet.

Marinated Grilled Butterflied Leg of Lamb

PROTEINS/FATS AND VEGGIES: LEVEL ONE

SERVES 10 TO 12

Spring is the season for lamb, one of my all-time favorite foods. This simple preparation with rosemary and garlic brings out the phenomenal taste of the lamb. The leg of lamb is a great meal for serving a larger group. Try it with my Baked Caramelized Onions (page 179).

6 garlic cloves, chopped
3 tablespoons chopped fresh rosemary
2 tablespoons salt
Freshly ground black pepper

3 tablespoons olive oil
1 7- to 8-pound leg of spring lamb (have your butcher debone and butterfly)
Juice of 1½ lemons

Preheat the grill to high heat.

In a small dish, mix together the chopped garlic, rosemary, salt, pepper to taste, and olive oil.

Place the deboned lamb in a roasting pan and rub all over on both sides with the garlic-olive oil mixture. Squeeze the juice from the lemons all over the lamb.

Let marinate at least 1 hour. (It's best if you marinate overnight so the flavors take hold. For overnight, place the lamb in a nonmetallic container covered with plastic wrap and refrigerate. Make sure to take the meat out and let it sit at room temperature for about 30 minutes before you grill it.)

Place the lamb on the hot grill and sear on each side for 5 to 7 minutes. This seals all the good juices inside.

Turn the heat down to medium and cook, turning often, for another 35 to 40 minutes. (If the grill has a cover, close it during cooking to roast the insides.)

Check for doneness by cutting into the thickest part of the meat. For medium, the lamb will be pink in the center. Return to the grill, if necessary. When done to your liking, remove from the grill and let stand for 10 minutes before carving. Carve into thin delicious slices and serve immediately.

Flattened Pan-Fried Pork Chops

PROTEINS/FATS AND VEGGIES: LEVEL ONE

SERVES 8

I love pounded chops. They take on a crispy, tangy, pan-fried flavor because they are marinated first, then cooked hot and fast.

8 boneless pork chops, pounded
6 garlic cloves
3 tablespoons salt
2 tablespoons black peppercorns

8 tablespoons chopped fresh rosemary
Juice of 4 lemons
10 to 11 tablespoons olive oil
8 lemon wedges

Ask your butcher to pound the chops between butcher paper with a heavy mallet until they are about ¹/₂-inch thick.

Place the garlic, salt, peppercorns, and rosemary into a plastic freezer bag. Seal the bag, then roughly pound the seasonings with a mallet or the bottom of a frying pan until the herbs are coarsely ground. (Make sure not to pierce the bag or the oil we're about to add will seep out.) Open the bag and add the lemon juice and about 8 table-

spoons of olive oil. Add the chops, reaching your hand in to spread the mixture over both sides of each chop. Leave in a cool place for about 1 hour.

Place a large skillet over medium-high heat. When the pan is hot, add 2 to 3 tablespoons olive oil. Add as many chops as will fit in the pan and fry for 5 to 6 minutes on each side. Repeat with the remaining chops.

Serve with lemon wedges.

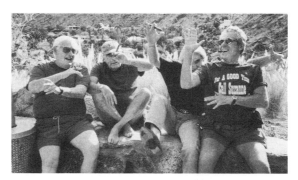

Alan and his pals at my 50th birthday party.

Braised Pork Chops with Purple Cabbage

PROTEINS/FATS AND VEGGIES: LEVEL ONE

SERVES 4

The pork drippings with the cabbage and port wine make a wonderful sauce for these chops.

8 ½-inch-thick pork chops
Salt and freshly ground black pepper
4 tablespoons olive oil
4 cups shredded purple cabbage

½ cup chicken stock (pages 123 and 125)
1 cup port wine
2 tablespoons balsamic vinegar
2 tablespoons (¼ stick) butter

Season the pork chops with salt and pepper on both sides.

Place a large skillet over medium-high heat. Add 2 tablespoons of the olive oil and the purple cabbage. Stir-fry until tender, about 5 minutes. Remove from the pan and set aside in a warm oven.

Place the skillet back over medium-high heat. Add the remaining 2 tablespoons of olive oil. Add the pork chops and cook for 5 to 6 minutes per side. Remove the chops from the pan and set aside with the cabbage. Add the stock, wine, and balsamic vinegar to the hot pan. Scrape all the bits from the bottom of the pan. Continue stirring until the sauce reduces by half. Turn off the heat and add the butter, 1 tablespoon at a time, until well combined.

Divide the cabbage among 4 plates. Top each with 2 pork chops.

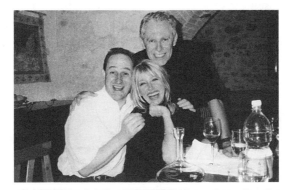

Alan and me having a fabulous Pork Chops with Purple Cabbage dinner at our friend Marco's vineyard in Tuscany.

Twelve-Hour Roast Pork

PROTEINS/FATS AND VEGGIES: LEVEL ONE

SERVES 15

I first tasted this at the River Cafe in London, the best restaurant in all of England. I believe I have re-created this recipe to be as good as theirs. It's perfect for a big casual party. I like to serve this in lettuce cups with Pico de Gallo (page 154) and sour cream. On Level Two I add whole wheat flour tortillas and serve it with Black Bean Chili (EGLW, page 143).

1 whole shoulder of pork with skin (7 to 9 pounds) (order this cut of meat in advance from your butcher)
12 garlic cloves, finely chopped
1 1.6-ounce bottle fennel seeds
Salt and freshly ground black pepper
8 small dried red chilies, crumbled

Juice of 6 lemons
4 tablespoons olive oil

PAN DRIPPINGS

1 14-ounce can chicken broth
Juice of 2 lemons

Preheat the oven to 450°F.

Score the entire skin of the shoulder by slicing deeply through the skin and into the meat. Continue scoring, making cuts ¼ inch apart from one another.

Place the garlic, fennel seeds, salt and pepper to taste, and chilies in a food processor. Pulse until all the seasonings are coarsely ground. (If you do not have a food processor, chop by hand on a cutting board.) Rub this mixture all over the skin of the pork and into the cut areas to cover all surfaces of the meat.

Place the shoulder on a rack in a roasting pan and roast for 30 minutes, or until the skin begins to crackle and brown. Loosen the shoulder from the bottom of the pan and pour half the lemon juice and 2 tablespoons of the olive oil over the pork.

Turn the oven temperature down to 250°F. and roast the pork for 12 to 18 hours. The pork becomes almost shredded, crispy on the outside and moist from the juices on the inside. It's ready when it is completely soft under the crisp skin. You can tell by pushing with your finger; the meat will give and might even fall off the bone. It will be cooked after 12 hours, but if you like it crispier, cook it for closer to 18 hours. Baste occasionally with the remaining lemon juice and olive oil.

Serve each person some of the crisp skin along with the meat.

For delicious pan drippings, remove the meat from the pan. Pour off most of the fat, leaving about 3 tablespoons in the pan. Place the roasting pan with all the bits of meat stuck to the bottom on the stove over medium heat. Scrape the bits as the pan heats up. When the pan gets good and hot, add the can of chicken broth and the juice of 2 lemons. Deglaze the pan by scraping all the bits from the bottom of the pan. Let the juices and the broth reduce for about 5 minutes. Spoon the sauce over the meat.

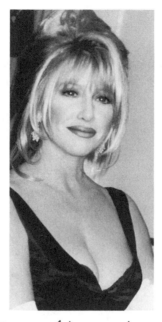

Moments before my show . . . Maybe I'm thinking about my 12-hour pork roast, which is in the oven ready to eat when I get home after the performance.

Pork Tenderloin with Sage

SERVES 4

Pork tenderloin is an elegant cut with a tender, fabulous flavor. Please don't overcook it! We were trained as kids only to eat pork cooked well done to guard against trichinosis. The trichinosis scare has been over for three decades! Enjoy this lovely meal prepared medium, with just a hint of pink in the center.

2 whole pork tenderloins
Salt and freshly ground black pepper
1 cup olive oil
Juice of 1 lemon
2 teaspoons finely chopped fresh sage (or 1
    teaspoon dried)

1 cup marsala wine or white wine
1 cup chicken stock (pages 123 and 125)
4 fresh sage leaves, finely chopped
2 tablespoons (¼ stick) butter

Preheat the oven to 350°F.

Place the pork tenderloins in a non-metallic container with the salt and pepper, olive oil, lemon juice, and chopped sage. Cover and refrigerate for at least 2 hours, turning after 1 hour.

Place a large skillet (ovenproof, if possible) over medium-high heat. Remove the tenderloins from the marinade and sear in the hot pan, turning frequently until browned all over.

If the skillet is ovenproof, place it in the oven and roast the tenderloins for 10 minutes. (If not, transfer the pork to a roasting pan, but use the skillet to make the sauce.)

When cooked, remove the pork from the skillet and set aside. Place the skillet over high heat. When hot, add the marsala wine. Cook until the steam evaporates. Add the chicken stock and the fresh chopped sage leaves, scraping the bits off the bottom of the pan. Cook over high heat until the sauce reduces by half or more. Turn off the heat and stir in the butter. Season with salt and pepper.

Cut the tenderloins into ½-inch-thick strips on an angle. Arrange in a semicircle on a plate and serve with sauce.

FOURTEEN

Level Two Recipes

Congratulations on advancing to Level Two! You have healed your metabolism by releasing the stored sugar from your cells. You have found your ideal body weight and now your body can handle a few treats here and there without causing too much of a problem. With Level Two, your goal is to maintain your weight. It's less strict than Level One eating. As my son, Bruce, says, "Level Two is just eating." And he's right. You don't ever have to deny yourself anything. You just can't indulge yourself every time you have a craving, but you can do it often enough so that you never feel deprived. You can stray from Level One eating as much as your body can handle, so go ahead and try some of the luscious Level Two desserts I've included here, such as Chocolate Pots de Crème or Ginger Crème Brûlée, and

see how you feel. Just remember that it's all about moderation. If you have a Level One meal, then enjoy a Level Two dessert now and then. If you eat a Level Two meal, such as Spinach and Ricotta Ravioli, then skip the dessert that day.

In addition to the Level Two recipes, you will continue to use all your favorite Level One recipes. If you don't already have *Eat Great, Lose Weight,* pick up a copy and enjoy all the fabulous recipes in that book. Remember to listen to your body. You will know you are creating too many imbalances if you feel tired, start to crave sugar or carbohydrates, and if the pounds begin to creep back on. If you notice any of these symptoms, go back to Level One guidelines until you get your balance back. Stay on top of the beautiful, healthy, new you as you learn to Somersize for the rest of your life. Enjoy!

Oatmeal Pancakes with Blueberry Sauce

LEVEL TWO

SERVES 4

These pancakes are delicious and much easier on your system than pancakes made from white flour that are topped with maple syrup. Use a nonstick pan to eliminate or cut down on the amount of oil you need to cook the pancakes. This is predominantly a Carbo meal, only the egg white, oil, and the blueberries make it Level Two.

PANCAKES

3/4 cup rolled oats
3/4 cup whole-wheat pastry flour
2 teaspoons baking powder
1/2 teaspoon baking soda
1/2 teaspoon salt
1 1/2 cups nonfat milk
1 large egg white, beaten

Mix all the dry ingredients together. Add the milk and beaten egg white and stir until combined.

Heat a nonstick griddle. Spray with cooking oil, then pour about 1/4 cup batter onto the griddle. When the pancakes bubble on the edges, slide a spatula under them and flip.

BLUEBERRY SAUCE

2 cups fresh blueberries or 1 package frozen
1 teaspoon fresh lemon juice
1/2 cup nonfat yogurt, optional (for a creamier sauce)

For the blueberry sauce, combine all the ingredients in a blender or food processor until smooth and well combined. (Strain through a sieve if you like a smooth sauce.) Drizzle the sauce over the pancakes and serve immediately.

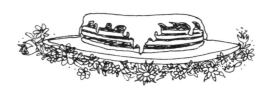

Lentil Salad

SERVES 2

Every year Alan and I vacation in St. Tropez, the heart of Provence, France. Placed on the table as a starter is always a bowl of freshly cooked tiny Le Puy lentils with chopped onions, olive oil, lemon, and salt and pepper. Try this. It's a satisfying and delicious lunch or main course if you are looking for a carbohydrate option. Only the addition of olive oil makes it Level Two. Omit the oil and you can eat it on Level One. It is simple, delicious, and healthy.

1 cup Le Puy lentils (I get mine at Trader Joe's in Southern California. They are also available from the Dean & Deluca catalog, 1-800-221-7714.)

Salt and freshly ground black pepper

1 cup chopped red (or Vidalia or Maui) onion

1 small bottle extra-virgin olive oil

2 to 3 lemons, cut into wedges

In a medium stockpot, put 4 to 6 cups water with the lentils and 1 tablespoon of salt. (The water should cover the lentils by 1 inch.) Bring to a boil for 20 to 25 minutes. Taste at 20 minutes for doneness; they should be soft but not mushy. When finished cooking, drain the lentils in a colander and set aside to cool.

Pour the cooled lentils into your prettiest country serving bowl. Also on the table arrange small separate bowls with chopped onion, olive oil, lemon wedges, and salt and pepper.

Let each person prepare their lentils according to taste. Some people like more onions than others. Do not skimp on the oil and lemons. Salt liberally and add freshly ground pepper.

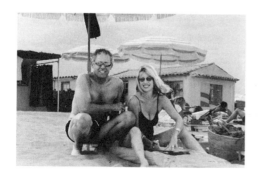

Alan and me enjoying the beach at St. Tropez. We will be having the Lentil Salad for lunch later on.

Pumpkin Soup with Roasted Shallots and Sage

SERVES 4 TO 6

This Level Two soup is the perfect holiday soup. It is much more exciting with fresh pumpkin, but canned will work if fresh is not available.

1 small pumpkin, about 5 pounds (or 2 29-ounce cans if fresh pumpkin is not available)
4 tablespoons olive oil
6 tablespoons (¾ stick) unsalted butter
2 medium onions, finely chopped
2 garlic cloves, peeled and minced

4 to 6 cups chicken stock (pages 123 and 125)
Salt and freshly ground black pepper
9 shallots, peeled and halved lengthwise
20 fresh sage leaves
2 cups vegetable oil

Preheat the oven to 350° F.

Quarter and seed the pumpkin. Rub the flesh with olive oil and bake on a baking sheet for 30 minutes. Set aside to cool.

Melt 4 tablespoons of butter in a heavy stockpot over medium heat. Cook the onions in the butter until translucent, about 7 minutes. Add the garlic and cook 1 minute longer. Meanwhile, scrape the flesh from the pumpkin and add to the onions. Cook for about 5 minutes.

Add 4 cups of chicken stock to the pot and simmer for 30 minutes. If you have a hand mixer, like the Braun hand mixer, you can place it right in the soup pot to puree the soup. Otherwise, transfer the soup to a blender or food processor and puree until smooth. Then return it to the pot. If necessary, thin with the remaining stock. Season with salt and pepper. Set the soup aside and keep it warm.

Melt the remaining butter in a small pan over medium heat and cook the shallots until golden and tender, about 15 minutes.

Fry the sage leaves in the vegetable oil until crisp. Drain on paper towels. Garnish each serving with 3 shallot halves and 3 sage leaves.

Fennel Soup with Ricotta Whole-Wheat Bruschetta

LEVEL TWO

SERVES 6

Alan and I first tasted this fabulous soup on a trip to Tuscany. The subtle combination of flavors makes this soup divine.

4 medium fennel bulbs
4 cups chicken stock (pages 123 and 125)
Salt and freshly ground black pepper
6 slices of crusty whole-wheat bread

1 garlic clove
12 tablespoons skim milk ricotta cheese
Extra-virgin olive oil
Freshly grated Parmesan cheese

To make the soup, slice a few of the feathery leaves from the tops of the fennel and set aside. Cut the stems off the fennel, leaving just the bulb to work with. Cut off any brown part on the bottom of the bulb. Remove and discard any tough or bruised outer layers of the fennel bulb and slice the bulbs into ½-inch pieces.

Bring the chicken stock to a boil and add the fennel pieces. Cook until tender, about 20 minutes. Add a few chopped fennel leaves and season with salt and pepper.

To make the ricotta whole-wheat bruschetta, grill or toast the whole-wheat bread slices. While still hot, rub the toast with a raw garlic clove. Spread 2 tablespoons ricotta cheese over each piece of toast and place a piece in each soup bowl.

Spoon the cooked fennel pieces over the bread, then ladle in some of the stock. Drizzle olive oil over each bowl. Season with pepper and Parmesan cheese and serve immediately.

Parsnip Garlic Ravioli with Mushroom Ragout

SERVES 2

This is a spectacular vegetarian meal. The ravioli are so light because they are made from wonton wrappers, which are available in the ethnic section of most grocery stores. I cooked this for Barry Manilow one evening and he flipped over it! It is Level Two because of the oil and butter in the ragout with the wonton wrappers and parsnip, which are carbohydrates.

MUSHROOM RAGOUT

2 tablespoons olive oil
2 medium onions, thinly sliced
1 tablespoon butter
1 pound portobello mushrooms, thinly
    sliced
3/4 pound white mushrooms, thinly sliced
3 garlic cloves, minced
1 teaspoon chopped fresh sage leaves

Salt and freshly ground black pepper
1 28- to 32-ounce can whole tomatoes,
    drained, coarsely chopped, juice reserved

RAVIOLIS

1 package 30 whole-wheat wonton
    wrappers, defrosted
1 recipe Parsnip Puree with Roasted Garlic
    (page 234)

For the mushroom ragout, in a large heated skillet, add the olive oil and sliced onions. Cook over medium heat for 10 minutes, until the onions are browned and caramelized, about 15 minutes. Stir often. Add the butter and stir until melted. Add all the mushrooms, garlic, sage, and salt and pepper to taste. Sauté, stirring constantly, for about 15 minutes, or until the mushroom liquid is evaporated. Stir in the tomatoes and reserved juice. Cook uncovered for 30 minutes. Stir occasionally.

For the raviolis, take each individual wonton wrapper and mound 1 level tablespoon of filling in the center. Brush the edges of the wrapper with water and fold the wrapper in half to form a triangle. Press securely on the edges to force out air. Finish the same process with the remaining wrappers. Place on a cookie sheet lightly floured with whole-wheat flour and cover with a light kitchen towel. Refrigerate until ready to use.

Cook the ravioli in a large pot of boiling water for approximately 5 minutes, or until they rise to the surface and are tender. Do not let the water boil vigorously once the ravioli have been added.

Immediately transfer the ravioli to serving plates. Top with mushroom ragout and serve.

Roasted Vegetable Sandwiches

LEVEL TWO

MAKES 24 FINGER SANDWICHES

These roasted vegetable sandwiches were a big hit at my granddaughter's christening. Another wonderful treat, thanks to Ken Brown.

1 zucchini, thinly sliced lengthwise
1 yellow squash, thinly sliced lengthwise
1 bell pepper, seeded and cut into quarters
2 tablespoons extra-virgin olive oil
1/4 cup balsamic vinegar

2 teaspoons kosher salt
Freshly ground black pepper
8 slices of whole-grain bread
1/2 cup Roasted Vegetable Dip (page 153)
8 ounces goat cheese, crumbled

Lay the vegetables out in a single layer on paper towels and sprinkle with salt. Let the vegetables sweat for 15 minutes before tossing with the oil, vinegar, kosher salt, and pepper.

Lightly grill the vegetables on a hot grill on both sides. Lightly grill the slices of bread, until barely charred. Spread the Roasted Vegetable Dip on the bread, then layer the grilled vegetables on 4 slices. Sprinkle on the goat cheese, then top with the remaining bread slices.

Cut each sandwich in half. Then cut each half into 3 triangles to make finger sandwiches.

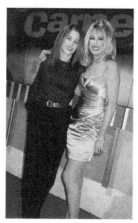

My talented stepdaughter Leslie and me. She always designs my beautiful dresses for Candid Camera.

Penne Pasta with Green Beans and Feta Cheese

LEVEL TWO

SERVES 4 TO 6 AS A SIDE DISH

My friend Ken Brown, the owner of Urban Epicuria, made his penne pasta recipe with whole-grain pasta for Violet's christening. It's still Level Two because it has oil and feta cheese. When you don't have time to make it yourself, there's nothing like having Ken around the corner.

½ pound whole-grain penne
½ pound string beans, cut into bite-size
   pieces
1 red bell pepper, cut into thin strips
¼ cup red wine vinegar
2 teaspoons fresh lemon juice
⅓ cup extra-virgin olive oil

2 tablespoons chopped parsley
2 teaspoons dried oregano
2 teaspoons kosher salt
½ pound crumbled feta cheese
½ cup kalamata olives (optional)
Freshly ground black pepper

Cook the pasta according to the package instructions until al dente (cooked through but not mushy).

Blanch the green beans by placing them in salted boiling water for approximately 3 minutes. Immediately immerse in ice water to halt the cooking process.

In a large bowl, toss the pasta and green beans with the remaining ingredients and mix well.

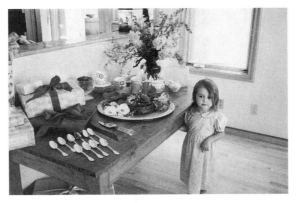

Camelia is eyeing the desserts at this tea.

Spinach and Ricotta Ravioli with Candied Tomato Sauce

LEVEL TWO

SERVES 4

I make these ravioli with whole-wheat wonton wrappers. It makes the process a lot faster and they are delicate and delicious. The sauce is made from pureeing the Candied Tomato recipe in Eat Great, Lose Weight, *or you may use your favorite tomato sauce.*

RAVIOLI

15 ounces nonfat ricotta cheese

½ pound fresh spinach, chopped, then steamed for 3 minutes

3 shallots, finely chopped

½ cup freshly grated Parmesan cheese

2 teaspoons finely chopped fresh basil (or 1 teaspoon dried)

1 tablespoon finely chopped parsley (or ½ tablespoon dried)

Salt and freshly ground black pepper

1 package (30) whole-wheat wonton wrappers

1 recipe Candied Tomato sauce (page 76 in *EGLW*)

To make the filling, place the ricotta, steamed spinach, shallots, Parmesan, basil, parsley, and salt and pepper in a mixing bowl. Stir until well combined.

To make the raviolis, place a single square wonton wrapper on a cutting board. Have a small glass of water standing by. Place a teaspoon of filling just off the center of the wrapper. To seal the ravioli, dip your finger in the water and wet the bottom two edges of the wonton. Fold the wonton in half to form a triangle. Gently press the edges together to force out air. Place in a single layer on a cookie sheet lightly floured with whole-wheat flour and cover with a light kitchen towel. (You can also place them in freezer bags, separating the layers with parchment paper. They will keep in the freezer for up to 3 months.)

When ready to cook, bring a large pot of salted water to a boil. Add the raviolis, one at a time, by carefully dropping them into the water. The raviolis are done shortly after they rise to the surface, or in about 5 minutes. Remove with a slotted spoon and place in individual serving bowls.

Top with a spoonful of Candied Tomato sauce and a sprinkle of Parmesan cheese.

For Level One

Eliminate the Parmesan cheese and make sure your pasta sauce has no oil in it.

Parsnip Puree with Roasted Garlic

LEVEL TWO

SERVES 4

Parsnips are a Funky Food, but still lower in sugar than potatoes. For Level Two you can enjoy this yummy side dish with a Pro/Fats and Veggies meal without creating a large imbalance.

2 garlic cloves
2 tablespoons olive oil
1 pound parsnips

4 ounces cream cheese, softened
Salt and freshly ground black pepper

Preheat the oven to 350°F.

To roast the garlic, put the cloves into a small pan with the olive oil. Roast in the oven for 30 minutes or sauté on top of the stove for 15 minutes.

To cook the parsnips, wash and peel the parsnips. Cut into 1-inch pieces and put into a 2-quart saucepan with just enough water to cover them. Cover and cook until tender, approximately 15 minutes.

Drain off the water and mash the parsnips with the cream cheese and roasted garlic. Season with salt and pepper.

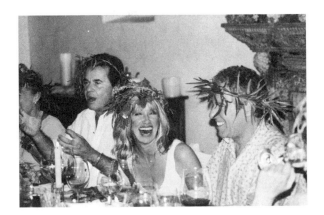

Kari (next to Dick) and Dick Clark, me, and Alan having fun around the dinner table at our desert home.

Baked Stuffed Eggplants
LEVEL TWO

SERVES 4

The additional olive oil and cheese mixed with the cannellini beans send this predominantly Carbos and Veggies meal into Level Two.

2 1-pound eggplants
¼ cup olive oil
Salt and freshly ground black pepper
1 medium onion, thinly sliced
1 garlic clove, minced

1 cup cooked or canned cannellini beans
3 ripe plum tomatoes, diced
1 teaspoon chopped fresh basil
2 fresh sage leaves, finely chopped
¼ cup grated Romano cheese

Preheat the oven to 400°F.

Cut the eggplants in half lengthwise. Make a couple of X's in the flesh of the eggplants for better olive oil penetration. Rub with a little of the olive oil and season with salt and pepper. Place cut side down in a baking dish and bake for 20 minutes.

In the meantime, place a skillet over medium-high heat. Add about 3 tablespoons olive oil and the onion. Sauté the onion until it becomes golden brown and begins to caramelize, about 15 minutes.

Add the garlic and cook 1 minute longer. Add the cooked beans, diced tomatoes, and herbs. Season with salt and pepper. Sauté for 2 minutes more, then remove from the heat.

When the eggplants have finished baking, turn them over, flesh side up, and top with the tomato and bean mixture. Place them back in the oven and bake for another 10 minutes.

Sprinkle with the grated Romano cheese and serve immediately.

Susie's Eggplant Manicotti
LEVEL TWO

SERVES 8

My friend Susie is a fabulous cook. Everything she makes elicits Mmmmm's. *She tells me, "I look for dishes that are good for entertaining." That way she can serve her guests three-course dinners that appear effortless. The following recipe is a mouthwatering first course. There are a lot of steps, but as Susie says, "I make the sauce ahead of time and freeze it." This is Level Two because there are carrots in the sauce, but you can easily replace Susie's sauce with another tomato sauce without carrots to enjoy this on Level One. I wanted to keep her recipe exactly as she makes it so it has to be a Level Two.*

FILLING

1 cup ricotta
$^1/_8$ cup grated Parmesan cheese
1 egg yolk
Salt and freshly ground black pepper
Freshly grated nutmeg
$^3/_4$ pound fresh spinach, washed and
    stemmed

EGGPLANTS

2 large eggplants
Olive oil

SAUCE

2 pounds tomatoes, washed and quartered
1 cup carrots, chopped
1 cup celery, chopped
$^3/_4$ cup onion, chopped
$^1/_4$ cup heavy cream
1 bunch of fresh basil leaves, cut into
    julienne

Preheat the oven to 350°F.

For the tomato sauce, cook the tomatoes in a large saucepan over low heat until the juice is released, about 10 minutes. Add the carrots, celery, and onion.

Simmer over low heat for about an hour, or until most of liquid has boiled away. Cool slightly and puree in a food processor or blender. Return to the pan over low heat and reduce by about a third. Stir in the

heavy cream and simmer 10 to 15 minutes or freeze at this point.

Peel the eggplants and slice lengthwise into $^1/_8$-inch-thick pieces. Place the slices in a colander and sprinkle them with salt. Let sit for about 30 minutes. Rinse very well, then pat the slices dry.

Lightly oil a cookie sheet. Place the eggplant slices in a single layer and lightly brush with oil. Bake for 20 minutes. The eggplant will become soft. Don't overcook the slices or they will become brittle and won't work for this recipe.

In a mixing bowl, combine the ricotta, Parmesan, egg yolk, salt and pepper, and grated nutmeg.

Place the spinach in a covered steamer basket over boiling water and steam for 3 minutes. Drain well, then chop and stir into the ricotta mixture. Set aside in the refrigerator.

To assemble the manicotti, place 1 table-spoon of ricotta filling near the edge of each slice of eggplant. Roll up and place on a lightly greased cookie sheet, forming manicotti-like tubes. (Note: These tubes can be made in advance and refrigerated overnight.)

Bake at 325°F. for 20 to 30 minutes.

For final assembly, spoon a bit of sauce on individual serving plates and top with 3 or 4 rolled, baked eggplant manicotti. Spoon on more sauce and garnish with basil. Serve immediately.

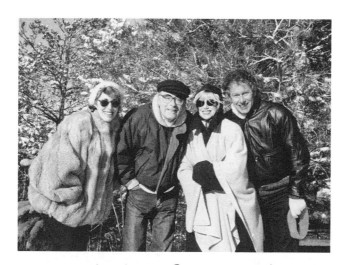

My dear friend Susie, her husband Arthur, me, and Alan. Four great friends enjoying the Canadian snow at their house.

Chocolate Pots de Crème

LEVEL TWO

SERVES 6 TO 8

These little pots are filled with the most creamy, velvety French chocolate pudding you've ever tasted. It's most special when served in "pot de crème" pots, which are little porcelain pots with lids. Of course, you may also use individual ½ cup ovenproof ramekins.

2 cups heavy cream
4 ounces dark chocolate
6 large egg yolks

2 tablespoons sugar
Pinch of salt
1½ teaspoons vanilla

Preheat the oven to 325°F. Place 1½ cups of the cream in a heavy small saucepan over low heat. Place the remaining ½ cup cream and the chocolate in the top of a large double boiler over hot water on medium heat.

In a mixing bowl, lightly stir the yolks just to mix—do not beat until foamy.

When the cream is scalded (a slight skin will form on the top), stir in the sugar and salt and remove from the heat.

Stir the chocolate mixture with a small wire whisk until perfectly smooth. Turn off the heat and very gradually add the hot cream to the chocolate, stirring constantly to keep the mixture smooth. Then gradually stir the chocolate mixture into the yolks and stir in the vanilla.

Return the mixture to the top of the double boiler over hot water on low heat and cook, stirring constantly with a rubber spatula, for 3 minutes.

Pour the mixture through a fine strainer into a pitcher. Then pour it into the individual ramekins or pots de crème cups, leaving a bit of headroom.

Place the cups in a shallow baking pan. Pour in hot water to about half the depth of the cups. Place the lids on top of the cups, or if you have used ramekins, place a cookie sheet over the top.

Bake for 22 minutes. The custard will look a little soft, but it will become firmer as it chills. It is best if it is still slightly creamy in the center when it is served. Remove the cups from the water and place on a rack to cool. Then refrigerate for a few hours. Serve with a spoonful of freshly whipped cream.

YUMMY!

Berry Confetti Cobbler

LEVEL TWO

SERVES 8

This berry cobbler is a snap to make and unbelievably great. Use whatever berries you have on hand. I made this with frozen wild blueberries and boysenberries and it was incredible. I don't top it with any added sugar, just a sprinkling of phyllo dough thinly sliced into a pile of confetti-like strips. It makes this dessert relatively low in sugar and great for Level Two. Serve it warm with a spoonful of whipped cream or vanilla ice cream. Heavenly.

2 tablespoons cornstarch
¼ cup orange juice
⅓ to ½ cup sugar (depending on the sweetness of the berries)
6 cups mixed berries (fresh or frozen)

1 package whole-wheat phyllo dough
3 tablespoons unsalted butter, melted

Preheat the oven to 450° F.

Mix the cornstarch and orange juice until smooth. Add the sugar and blend until well combined. Gently toss the berries with the mixture and let sit for about 15 minutes.

Take the phyllo dough out of the package. Unroll the dough and remove the piece of paper in the center. Roll the phyllo back up and place on a chopping block. Starting at one end, slice the phyllo dough into thin strips. You will only need about one quarter of the package. (Reinsert the piece of paper before returning the phyllo to the freezer.) Separate the sliced layers of phyllo to make a small pile of "confetti."

Pour the berries with their juice into a 9 × 11-inch baking dish. Sprinkle the confetti evenly over the top. Drizzle all over with the melted butter.

Bake at 450° F. for 10 minutes. Turn down the heat to 350° F. and bake another 45 minutes, until the juices are thick and bubbly. Let cool at least 10 minutes.

Spoon the cobbler into bowls and serve as is, or with a spoonful of whipped cream or vanilla ice cream.

Crème Brûlée

LEVEL TWO

SERVES 8

Crème Brûlée is creamy little individual custards topped with a thin hard layer of caramelized sugar. It's one of my favorite things.

Unsalted butter
9 large egg yolks
$\frac{1}{3}$ cup plus 8 tablespoons sugar

$1\frac{1}{2}$ cups heavy cream
1 vanilla bean, split lengthwise

Lightly butter 8 5-inch heatproof rame-kins (little soufflé dishes).

Fill a large bowl with ice cubes. Set aside.

In a medium heatproof bowl, whisk together the egg yolks and $\frac{1}{3}$ cup of sugar. Set aside.

In heavy medium saucepan, combine the cream and the vanilla bean with its scrapings. Bring just to a boil over low heat.

Place the bowl with the egg yolks over a pan of simmering water and continue to whisk vigorously until the mixture becomes a very pale yellow and feels hot to the touch. Remove the bowl from the heat and whisk in the boiling cream. Transfer the bowl back over the saucepan, but do not turn on the heat. Whisk the mixture occasionally until it thickens, 5 to 10 minutes.

When the mixture thickens, place the bowl in the larger bowl filled with ice cubes. Whisk occasionally until cool. Strain into a clean bowl.

Spoon the custard into the prepared ramekins and refrigerate, covered, until firm, about 2 hours.

When ready to serve, sprinkle 1 tablespoon sugar evenly over the top of each serving and caramelize with a propane torch or set under a broiler until the sugar browns.

Raspberry Crème Brûlée

Using 2 cartons of fresh raspberries, place as many raspberries as will fit side by side in the bottom of each ramekin.

Proceed with Crème Brûlée instructions above.

Ginger Crème Brûlée

SERVES 8

This crème brûlée has the exotic addition of ginger. It's perfect after an Asian meal.

Unsalted butter
9 large egg yolks
$1/3$ cup plus 8 tablespoons sugar

$1\frac{1}{2}$ cups heavy cream
4 or 5 slices of fresh ginger, peeled and
    blanched in boiling water for 30 seconds

Lightly butter 8 5-inch heatproof rame-kins (little soufflé dishes).

Fill a large bowl with ice cubes. Set aside.

In a medium heatproof bowl, whisk together the egg yolks and $1/3$ cup of sugar. Set aside.

In a heavy medium saucepan, combine the cream and the ginger. Bring just to a boil over low heat.

Place the bowl with the egg yolks over a pan of simmering water and continue to whisk vigorously until the mixture becomes a very pale yellow and feels hot to the touch. Remove the bowl from the heat and whisk in the boiling cream. Transfer the

bowl back over the saucepan but do not turn on the heat. Whisk the mixture occasionally until it thickens, 5 to 10 minutes.

When the mixture thickens, place the bowl in the larger bowl filled with ice cubes. Whisk occasionally until cool. Strain into a clean bowl.

Spoon the custard into the prepared ramekins and refrigerate, covered, until firm, about 2 hours.

When ready to serve, sprinkle 1 table-spoon sugar evenly over the top of each serving and caramelize with a propane torch or set under a broiler until the sugar browns.

Bruce's Cafe Legois

LEVEL TWO

SERVES 4

When Bruce was a teenager he biked across France with his school. It was on this trip that he discovered the magnificent dessert Cafe Legois. It's still his favorite. He serves it in tall ice cream soda glasses.

CHOCOLATE SAUCE

6 ounces dark chocolate, broken up
³/4 cup heavy cream

1 pint good-quality coffee ice cream
   (Häagen-Dazs or Breyer's)
½ cup hot decaf espresso (or strong decaf
   coffee)

GARNISH

1 cup freshly whipped cream
Chocolate-covered decaf espresso beans
   (optional)

To make the chocolate sauce, place the broken-up chocolate in a bowl. Place the cream in a saucepan and bring to a boil. Add the hot cream to the chocolate and stir until all the lumps are gone.

Place 2 scoops of coffee ice cream in each glass. Pour a little hot decaf espresso over the top of each. Drizzle a little chocolate sauce over the top. Garnish with freshly whipped cream and a couple of chocolate-covered espresso beans, if you like. Serve immediately.

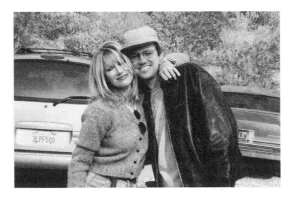

I love Bruce so much!

Strawberry Gratin

LEVEL TWO

SERVES 4

When the French have nothing prepared for dessert, they make gratin. It's simply fresh berries, covered with sour cream, then sprinkled with sugar and placed under the broiler. It's a perfect low-sugar Level Two dessert made with any kind of berries.

4 cups strawberries
2 cups sour cream
1 tablespoon granulated sugar

2 teaspoons vanilla
3 tablespoons brown sugar

Preheat the broiler.

Wash the strawberries and slice off the end with the stem. Place the berries, cut side down, sitting upright in a tart pan. Nuzzle them together, side by side, as many as will fit in the pan.

In a bowl, mix together the sour cream, granulated sugar, and vanilla. Pour over the berries. Sprinkle the brown sugar over the strawberries and broil for 3 to 5 minutes, until the top gets brown and crusty. Serve warm.

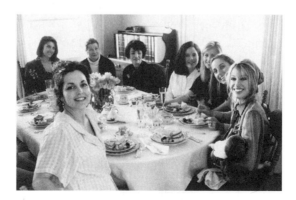

A very pregnant Caroline gives a tea for "the girls."

Mountain of Lemon Meringue Pie

MAKES 6 TO 8 SERVINGS

This pie is spectacular, with a mountain of meringue piled high. And my lemon curd filling is the best I've ever tasted, if I do say so myself.

WHOLE-WHEAT PASTRY CRUST

1 cup whole-wheat pastry flour
2 tablespoons sugar
½ teaspoon salt
6 tablespoons (¾ stick) butter, softened
1 large egg yolk
½ teaspoon vanilla
1 tablespoon fresh lemon juice

LEMON FILLING

3 tablespoons butter, softened
¼ cup honey
2 large eggs, lightly beaten
¼ cup fresh lemon juice
Grated zest of 2 lemons

MERINGUE

6 egg whites
¼ teaspoon cream of tartar
3 to 4 tablespoons sugar

Preheat the oven to 400°F. Butter and flour a 9-inch tart or pie pan.

To make the crust, in a mixing bowl, combine the flour, sugar, and salt. Add the softened butter and work together with your fingertips or a pastry blender. Make a well in the center of the mixture (push the flour mixture to the sides of the bowl) and add the egg yolk, vanilla, and lemon juice. Mix the wet ingredients together with your fingertips and slowly incorporate the dry ingredients until the dough forms a ball and no longer adheres to your hands. Cover with wax paper and refrigerate for at least 30 minutes.

Roll out the chilled dough on a floured board (see Note). Place the dough in the pie or tart pan, poke with a fork in several places, and bake for 7 to 10 minutes, until golden brown.

To make the filling, blend the butter and honey in a double boiler (or a heatproof bowl over a saucepan of boiling water). When well combined, mix in the eggs, stirring constantly. Add the lemon juice and zest. Continue stirring until the custard thickens and coats the back of a wooden spoon.

Fill the crust with the lemon pie filling. Set aside until the filling is set while you make the meringue.

Preheat the oven to 375°F.

Beat the egg whites with the cream of tartar until fluffy. Continue beating and gradually add the sugar. Beat for 5 to 8 minutes, until stiff peaks form.

Smooth the meringue over the filling, covering the filling completely. Spoon the rest of the meringue onto the center of the pie. Using a spatula, draw the meringue upward so it resembles a mountain of meringue.

Bake for 7 to 10 minutes, or until the meringue is golden brown. Serve at room temperature. Do not chill.

Note

Sometimes whole-wheat dough can be difficult to roll out. If you have a problem, simply press the dough with your fingertips into the pie or tart pan.

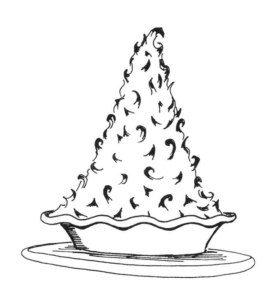

Cappuccino Chocolate Chunk Cheesecake

SERVES 8

This cheesecake has the mellow flavor of coffee with chunks of dark chocolate. Oh, my. I use about half the amount of sugar you'll find in most cheesecake recipes and I think it's sweet and delicious. You can add a little extra if you like it sweeter. I don't like to use artificial sweetener, but this recipe also works with 12 packets of sweetener instead of the sugar.

2 packages (8 ounces each) cream cheese
1/2 cup sugar
3 large eggs
1 1/2 teaspoons vanilla
1/4 teaspoon salt
1/4 cup decaf espresso or strong decaf coffee

GARNISH

4 ounces dark chocolate, broken into small
 pieces
3 cups sour cream
Chocolate-covered decaf coffee beans

Preheat the oven to 350°F.

In a large mixing bowl, beat the cream cheese and sugar until very smooth, about 3 minutes. Add the eggs, one at a time, beating well after each addition. Add the vanilla, salt, and decaf espresso and chocolate when using. Beat in the sour cream until just blended.

Grease a 9-inch springform pan with 2 1/2-inch sides and line the bottom with greased parchment or wax paper. Wrap the outside of the pan with a double layer of heavy-duty foil to prevent seepage.

Pour the batter into the pan. Sprinkle broken chocolate bits on top of the batter. Set the pan in a large roasting pan and surround with 1 inch of very hot water. Bake for 45 minutes. Turn off the oven without opening the door and let the cake cool 1 hour.

Remove to a rack and cool to room temperature, about 1 hour. Cover with plastic wrap and refrigerate overnight. Unmold the cake onto a plate and garnish with chocolate-covered decaf coffee beans.

Almond Chocolate Torte

SERVES 8-10

This cake is simply divine. It's made without any added flour and a relatively low amount of sugar. Serve it with freshly whipped cream and oh, my. Yummmmmmmm!

1½ cups whole blanched almonds
8 ounces dark chocolate, broken into
   pieces

1 cup (2 sticks) unsalted butter, softened
⅓ cup sugar
6 large eggs, separated

Preheat the oven to 400° F.

Butter an 8-inch round springform pan. Line the bottom with buttered wax paper.

Coarsely grind the almonds in a food processor. Add the chocolate and grind until the chocolate is broken into small pieces.

Cream the butter and sugar together with an electric mixer until light and pale. Add the egg yolks one by one, mixing well between each addition. Then add the chocolate and nut mixture, blending until just combined.

In a separate bowl, beat the egg whites until they form soft peaks. Using a spatula, fold one quarter of the egg whites into the chocolate mixture with large circular motions. Now take this chocolate mixture and fold it into the remaining egg whites.

Pour the batter into the prepared pan. Bake for 45 minutes, or until a toothpick comes out clean.

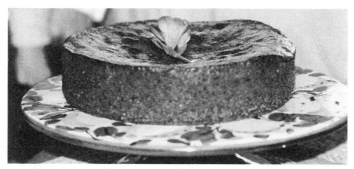

I made this torte for one of our Sunday summer family dinners at the beach.

Frozen Chocolate Mousse Pie with Chocolate Mint Leaves

LEVEL TWO

SERVES 8

When you freeze this chocolate mousse in a pie pan, it makes a crustless pie with no flour and no added sugar (only the sugar found in the dark chocolate). I like to decorate the edge with Chocolate Mint Leaves.

12 ounces dark chocolate, broken up
¾ cup boiling water
8 large eggs, separated
4 tablespoons Grand Marnier (orange-flavored liqueur)
¼ cup sugar or 3 packets artificial sweetener, if desired (optional)

GARNISH

1 pint heavy cream
1 teaspoon vanilla
Chocolate Mint Leaves (page 250)

Butter a 9-inch pie pan.

Place the chocolate in a blender or food processor and blend until reduced to a powder. Add the boiling water and blend until smooth. Then add the egg yolks and liqueur and blend until well combined. (If you prefer the mousse a little sweeter, add ¼ cup of sugar or 3 packets of artificial sweetener.)

In a separate bowl, beat the egg whites until they form stiff peaks. Using a large spatula, fold the chocolate mixture into the egg whites. Make large circular motions to blend thoroughly without deflating the egg whites.

Pour the mousse into the prepared pie pan and freeze for at least 4 hours before serving.

Before serving the pie, whip the cream with the vanilla until soft peaks form. (For sweetened whipped cream, add 1 tablespoon of sugar or 1 packet of artificial sweetener.) Decorate the edge of the pie with whipped cream and Chocolate Mint Leaves.

Decadent White Chocolate Cake

SERVES 8–10

This elegant, pound-like cake is the white chocolate version of my Decadent Chocolate Cake from Eat Great, Lose Weight. *Use a good-quality white chocolate—I prefer Valhrona. White chocolate chips do not work well because they are made with a lot of oil. For a beautiful decoration, dip one side of small leaves into melted white chocolate. Place them on a cookie sheet in the freezer. When they are set, peel off the leaves and place the white chocolate decorative leaves on the cake. Beautiful.*

CAKE

14 ounces white chocolate
22 tablespoons unsalted butter
8 large eggs, separated
½ cup sugar
⅔ cup whole-wheat pastry flour

GANACHE

8 ounces white chocolate, broken up
1¾ cup heavy cream

Preheat the oven to 350°F.

Butter and flour 2 9-inch round cake pans.

For the cake, melt the white chocolate and butter in a double boiler or a heatproof bowl placed over a saucepan of boiling water. Set aside to cool.

Beat the egg yolks until light and fluffy. Slowly add the sugar and continue beating until the mixture is pale yellow. Fold in the melted white chocolate. Sift the flour over the chocolate mixture until it just disappears.

In a separate bowl, whisk the egg whites until soft peaks form. Fold the beaten egg whites into the white chocolate mixture in 2 parts. Pour the batter into the prepared pan and tap on the counter to remove any air bubbles. Bake 20 to 30 minutes, until a toothpick comes out clean with a few flakes sticking to it.

For the ganache, place the white chocolate in a mixing bowl. Place the cream in a saucepan and bring to a boil. Add the hot cream to the white chocolate and stir until all lumps are gone. Let the ganache stand until it reaches room temperature, about an hour. Trim any uneven sections off the top of the cooled cakes so they will stack evenly. Place these cut sides together, securing them with a thin layer of ganache. Brush any crumbs off the stacked cakes and pour the remaining ganache over the top, spreading the top and sides evenly with a spatula. Chill the frosted cake until ready to serve.

Chocolate Mint Leaves

LEVEL TWO

MAKES APPROXIMATELY 30 LEAVES

These are great tasting and make wonderful decorations for any of my desserts. You can eat the mint leaves like they are, as little candies, or use them to decorate cakes or custards. I like to cascade the leaves down the side of the Decadent Chocolate Cake (EGLW, page 200). This also works well with white chocolate.

For this recipe, you will need parchment paper, a small unused paintbrush, and a rolling pin.

6 ounces dark chocolate

Melt the chocolate in a double boiler or a heatproof bowl set over a saucepan of simmering hot water, stirring constantly, making sure the chocolate does not get too warm. Remove the bowl from the heat and continue to stir until the chocolate is melted and smooth as silk.

Place a piece of parchment or wax paper on a cookie sheet. Place a rolling pin, covered with plastic wrap, on the paper.

Take a mint leaf by its stem and dip it

Clean dry mint leaves

into the chocolate. Place the leaf on the rolling pin to dry. Be sure you coat both sides of the mint leaf, then brush the stem with chocolate. Putting it on a rolling pin causes the leaf to dry with a natural curl to it.

Complete these steps with the remainder of the chocolate.

Put the leaves into the freezer to set. When dry and frozen, put them into a freezer bag and use as needed.

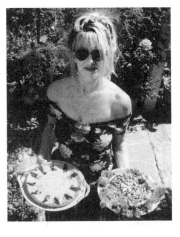

I love dessert, especially Somersized ones, right out of my oven.

Easy Ice Cream Coffee Treat

SERVES 4

There's nothing like dessert and coffee when you're sitting around with your loved ones. One of my notorious treats is a combination of the two. The hot coffee is poured over the ice cream, melting it into this yummy cappuccino cream dream. You'll feel like picking up the bowl and drinking every last drop. Pick up a pint of good-quality ice cream from the store, such as Häagen-Dazs or Breyer's All Natural Vanilla. Both are made without chemicals and preservatives.

8 small scoops of vanilla ice cream

12 tablespoons strong decaf coffee

Place 2 scoops of the ice cream into 4 small bowls (silver ice cream dishes are great). Pour 3 tablespoons of the hot coffee over the top of each and serve immediately.

Caramel Sauce

LEVEL TWO

SERVES 4

Enjoy this delicious caramel sauce drizzled over ice cream, cheesecake, or your favorite dessert. White grape juice is used as the sweetener, but it's still a form of sugar, so use this sauce sparingly.

1 cup white grape juice
1 tablespoon unsalted butter

1 tablespoon heavy cream

In a saucepan, cook the white grape juice over high heat until it reduces to about ¼ cup. Add the butter while stirring constantly. Add the heavy cream and remove from the heat.

When this sauce cools, it will have the consistency of caramel.

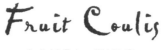

Fruit Coulis

MAKES ABOUT 1 ½ CUPS

A fruit coulis is a fruit puree used as a sauce for decorating desserts or covering dessert plates. There are several methods to do this. The outcome is the same—a smooth fruit puree thin enough to pour. You do not want seeds or lumps.

2 cups white grape juice

1½ cups fresh or frozen fruit of choice

Place the white grape juice in a medium saucepan over high heat. Reduce it to ½ cup. This will make a thick syrup.

Puree the fruit in a blender or food processor until smooth. Add the reduced grape juice, stirring to combine. Strain through a fine sieve to get rid of any seeds and skins. The sauce will be the perfect consistency for decorating plates and desserts. Keep the extra sauce in marked freezer bags. Whenever you need a dessert sauce, set a bag out to defrost. Then cut off a tiny corner of the freezer bag and squeeze out the coulis, using it like a pastry bag.

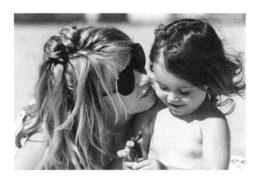

Me and Camelia at the beach.

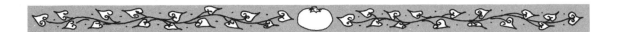

A Final Note

It is time to reflect now on all the wonderful changes that can occur in your life because of Somersizing. With your new figure and your improved health comes a renewed sense of self-confidence. You set out to achieve a goal, and you have attained it. You should be proud of yourself. Enjoy your meals, enjoy your new body, and enjoy knowing that you are giving your body the nutritious foods it needs to thrive and ward off disease. Somersizing has truly been a liberating experience for me. I am finally in control of my weight rather than my weight being in control of me. I hope that in sharing my program and my recipes with you, your life has been enhanced in some way, either through losing a few pounds or by learning some new tricks in the kitchen.

My favorite part about putting together this book was reading all the success stories from people just like you. I can't tell you how gratifying it is for me to hear about the weight you've lost and how you've learned to cook some fabulous new recipes. Please write to me and let me know how you are doing on the program. I would love to hear from you. And if you like, pass along any good recipes of your own! You can send them to me c/o Crown Publishers, Inc., 201 East 50th Street, New York, New York 10022.

Congratulations, once again . . . it's been a pleasure Somersizing with you. Now go *Get Skinny on Fabulous Food!*

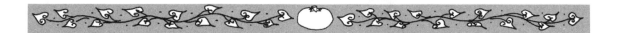

Reference Guide

Here is a complete list of all the foods available in each of the categories:

PRO/FATS

CHEESE
American
asiago
Babybel
bel paese
blue
Bonbel
Brie
buffalo mozzarella
Camembert
Cheddar
Colby
cottage cheese
cream cheese
farmer

feta
fontina
goat
gouda
Gruyère
Havarti
hoop
Jarlsberg
Limburger
mascarpone
Monterey jack
mozzarella
Muenster
Parmesan
pecorino

provolone
queso blanco
ricotta
Romano
Roquefort
string
Swiss

OTHER DAIRY
PRODUCTS
butter
cream
eggs
margarine
mayonnaise

sour cream

FISH
anchovy
bass
bluefish
bonito
burbot
carp
catfish
cod
eel
flatfish
flounder
gefilte fish

grouper
haddock
halibut
herring
mackerel
mahi-mahi
monkfish
ocean perch
orange roughy
pollack
pompano
red snapper
sablefish
salmon
sardine
sea bass
shark
smelt
snapper
sole

sturgeon
swordfish
trout
tuna
turbot
whitefish
wolf fish
yellowtail

MEAT
bacon
Canadian bacon
beef
bratwurst
bologna
capocollo
cold cuts
frog's legs
ham
hot dogs
lamb

pastrami
pepperoni
pork
prosciutto
rabbit
salami
sausage
veal
venison

OILS
chile oil
olive oil
peanut oil
safflower oil
sesame oil
vegetable oil

POULTRY
capon
chicken

Cornish game hen
duck
goose
guinea hen
pheasant
quail
squab
turkey

SEAFOOD
abalone
caviar
clams
crab
crayfish
lobster
mussels
octopus
scallops
shrimp
squid

CARBOS

BEANS
adzuki beans
anasazi beans
black beans
black-eyed peas
cannellini beans
fava beans
garbanzo beans
great northern
    beans
green peas
kidney beans
lentils
lima beans
mung beans
navy beans

pinto beans
red beans
split peas
white beans

BREADS,
BAGELS,
CRACKERS,
HOT CEREALS,
COLD CEREALS,
OR PASTA
MADE FROM
WHOLE
GRAINS
amaranth
barley
bran

brown rice
buckwheat
durum wheat
farina
kamut
millet
oats
pumpernickel
rye
spelt
wheat

TABBOULEH

WHEAT GERM

PHYLLO
DOUGH

NONFAT
DAIRY
PRODUCTS
nonfat cottage
    cheese
nonfat milk
nonfat ricotta
    cheese
nonfat sour cream
nonfat yogurt

RICE
brown rice
brown rice cakes
wild rice

VEGGIES

alfalfa sprouts
artichoke
arugula
asparagus
bamboo shouts
basil
bean sprouts
beet greens
bok choy
broccoli
brussels sprouts
cabbage
cauliflower
celery
chervil
chicory greens
chives
cilantro
clover sprouts
collard greens
crookneck squash

cucumber
daikon
dandelion greens
dill weed
eggplant
endive
escarole
fennel
garlic
ginger
green beans
horseradish
jicama
kale
kohlrabi
leeks
lettuce
   Boston or bibb
   iceberg
   limestone
   red oak

romaine
mushrooms
mustard greens
okra
onion
parsley
peppers
   bell peppers
   cherry peppers
   chile peppers
   peperoncini
   piccalilli
   pickles (except
     sweet)
purslane
radicchio
radish
rhubarb
rosemary
sage
salsify

sauerkraut
shallots
snow peas
spinach
sugar snap peas
Swiss chard
tarragon
thyme
tomatillo
tomato
tomato (green)
turnip
turnip greens
watercress
wax beans
yard-long beans
yellow beans
zucchini

FRUIT

apples
apricots
Asian pear
berries
   blackberry
   blueberry
   boysenberry
   cranberry
   currant
   elderberry
   gooseberry
   mulberry
   ollalaberry
   raspberry

strawberry
cherimoya
cherry
crabapple
fig
grapefruit
grapes
guava
kiwi
kumquat
lemon
lime
loquat
lychee

mangoes
mandarin oranges
melons
   cantaloupe
   casaba
   Crenshaw
   honeydew
   orange flesh
   sharlyn
watermelon
nectarines
oranges
papaya
passion fruit

peaches
pears
persimmon
pineapple
plums
pomegranate
prickly pear
pommelo
quince
star fruit
tamarind
tangerine

YOUR ONE-PAGE REFERENCE GUIDE

For the first few days or weeks on the program, you might want to make a copy of this page and slip it into your purse or wallet. Somersizing will soon become second nature to you, but this summary will help remind you of the plan until you no longer need if for reference.

1. Eliminate all Funky Foods.
2. Eat Fruits alone, on an empty stomach.
3. Eat Proteins/Fats with Veggies.
4. Eat Carbos with Veggies and no fat.
5. Keep Proteins/Fats separate from Carbos.
6. Wait three hours between meals if switching from a Proteins/Fats meal to a Carbos meal, or vice versa.
7. Do not skip meals. Eat three meals a day, and eat until you feel satisfied and comfortably full.

PROTEINS AND FATS

Butter	Mayonnaise
Cheese	Meat
Cream	Oil
Eggs	Poultry
Fish	Sour cream

VEGGIES

Asparagus	Green beans
Broccoli	Lettuce
Cauliflower	Mushrooms
Celery	Spinach
Cucumber	Tomato
Eggplant	Zucchini

CARBOS

Beans	Whole-grain
Mustard	breads, cereals,
Nonfat milk	pastas
products	

FRUITS

Apples	Oranges
Berries	Papaya
Grapes	Peaches
Mangoes	Pears
Melons	Plums
Nectarines	

Eliminate Funky Foods

SUGAR

Beets	Maple syrup
Carrots	Molasses
Corn syrup	Sugar
Honey	

STARCHES

Bananas	Potatoes
Corn	Sweet potatoes
Pasta made from	White flour
semolina or	White rice
white flour	Winter squashes
Popcorn	

COMBO PROTEINS/FATS AND CARBOS

Avocados	Nuts
Coconuts	Olives
Liver	Tofu
Low-fat or	
whole milk	

CAFFEINE AND ALCOHOL

Alcoholic beverages
Caffeinated coffees, teas, and sodas
Cocoa

Bibliography

Anderson, K. M., W. P. Castelli, and D. Levy. "Cholesterol and Mortality: 30 Years of Follow-up from the Framingham Study," *JAMA* 257(1987): 2176–80.

Applegate, Liz. "Fats as Fuel? A Little More Fat in Your Diet May Help You on Your Next Run," *Runner's World* 29, no. 6 (June 1994): 24.

Atkins, Robert C. "Artificial Sugar: A Sweet and Dangerous Lure," *Dr. Atkins' Health Revelations* (April 1994): 1.

Brown, David. "Linkage of Breast Cancer, Dietary Fat Is Discounted," *The Washington Post* 119, no. 65 (February 8, 1996): A5 col 1.

Carlson, L. A., L. E. Bottiger, and P. E. Anfeldt. "Risk Factors for Myocardial Infarction in the Stockholm Prospective Study: A 14 year Follow-up Focusing on the Role of Plasma Triglycerides and Cholesterol," *Acta Med Scand* 206 (1979): 351–60.

Clark, Nancy. "Fat and Fiction: Dispelling the Myths About Fat in a Healthy Diet," *American Fitness* 15, no. 3 (May–June 1997): 59.

DeFronzo, R. A. "Insulin Secretion, Insulin Resistance, and Obesity." *Int J Obes* 6 (Suppl. 1) (1982): 72–82.

DeFronzo, R. A., and E. Ferrannini. "Insulin Resistance: A Multifaceted Syndrome Responsible for NIDDM, Obesity, Hypertension, Dyslipemia, and Atherosclerotic Cardiovascular Disease," *Diabetes Care* 14, no. 3 (March 1991): 173.

Fackelmann, K. "Hidden Hazards: Do High Blood Insulin Levels Foretell Heart Disease?" *Science News* 136 (September 16, 1989): 184.

Fontbonne, A. "Why Can High Insulin Levels Indicate a Risk Factor for Coronary Heart Disease?" *Diabetologia* 37 (1994): 953–5.

Grundy, Scott M. "Cholesterol and Coronary Disease," *JAMA* 256 (1986): 2849–58.

———. "Fats and Oil Consumption to Combat Metabolic Complications and Obesity," *American Journal of Clinical Nutrition* 67, no. 3 (March 1998): 5275.

Howe, Maggy. "Good Fats, Bad Fats," *Country Living* 21, no. 1 (January 1998): 50.

Jenkins, J. A., et al. "Starchy Foods and Glycemic Index," *Diabetes Care* 11, no. 2 (February 1998): 149.

Modann, M., H. Halkin, S. Almog, et al. "Hyperinsulinemia: A Link Between Hypertension, Obesity, and Glucose Intolerance," *J Clin Invest* 75 (1985): 809–17.

Page, Douglas. "Give Fat a Break," *Muscle and Fitness* 58, no. 5 (May 1997): 58.

Pollare, T., H. Lithell, and C. Berne. "Insulin Resistance Is a Characteristic Feature of Primary Hypertension Independent of Obesity," *Metabolism* 39 (1990): 167–74.

Raloff, Janet. "High Fat Diets Help Athletes Perform," *Science News* 149, no. 18 (May 4, 1996): 287.

Reaven, G. M. "Banting Lecture: Role of Insulin Resistance in Human Disease," *Diabetes* 37 (1988): 1595–1607.

Reaven, G. M., C. B. Hollenbeck, and Y-DI Chen. "Relationship Between Glucose Tolerance, Insulin Secretion, and Insulin Action in Non-Obese Individuals with Varying Degrees of Glucose Tolerance," *Diabetologia* 32 (1989): 52–55.

Reppert, Bertha, and Sharon Mikkelson.

"Stevia (Stevia rebaudiana 'honeyleaf')," *American Health and Herbs* (1998): 1–7.

Schechter, Steven. "Fat Intake Can Boost Weight Loss, If We Are Selective About Our Choices," *Better Nutrition* 59, no. 6 (June 1997): 26.

Schwarzbein, Diana, and Nancy Deville. *The Schwarzbein Principle.* California: Health Communications, Inc., 1999.

Shapiro, Laura. "In Sugar We Trust," *Newsweek* (July 13, 1998): 72.

Sowers, J. R., M. Nyby, N. Stern, F. Beck, S. Baron, R. Catania, and N. Vlachis. "Blood Pressure and Hormone Changes Associated with Weight Reduction in the Obese," *Hypertension* 4 (1982): 686–91.

Stout, Robert W. "Insulin and Atheroma Twenty Year Perspective." *Diabetes Care* 13, no. 6 (June 1990): 631.

Wingard, D. L., E. L. Barrett-Connor, and A. Ferrara. "Is Insulin Really a Heart Disease Risk Factor?" *Diabetes Care* 18 (1995): 1299–1304.

Zavaroni, I., et al. "Risk Factors for Coronary Artery Disease in Healthy Persons with Hyperinsulinemia and Normal Glucose Tolerance," *NEJM* 320 (March 16, 1989): 702.

Index

CONVERSION CHART
EQUIVALENT IMPERIAL AND METRIC MEASUREMENTS

American cooks use standard containers, the 8-ounce cup and a tablespoon that takes exactly 16 level fillings to fill that cup level. Measuring by cup makes it very difficult to give weight equivalents, as a cup of densely packed butter will weigh considerably more than a cup of flour. The easiest way therefore to deal with cup measurements in recipes is to take the amount by volume rather than by weight. Thus the equation reads:

1 cup = 240 ml = 8 fl. oz.   1/2 cup = 120 ml = 4 fl. oz.

It is possible to buy a set of American cup measures in major stores around the world.

In the States, butter is often measured in sticks. One stick is the equivalent of 8 tablespoons. One tablespoon of butter is therefore the equivalent to ½ ounce/15 grams.

SOLID MEASURES

U.S. and Imperial Measures		Metric Measures	
Ounces	Pounds	Grams	Kilos
1		28	
2		56	
3½		100	
4	¼	112	
5		140	
6		168	
8	½	225	
9		250	¼
12	¾	340	
16	1	450	
18		500	½
20	1¼	560	
24	1½	675	
27		750	¾
28	1¾	780	
32	2	900	
36	2¼	1000	1
40	2½	1100	
48	3	1350	
54		1500	1½
64	4	1800	
72	4½	2000	2
80	5	2250	2¼
90		2500	2½
100	6	2800	2¾

LIQUID MEASURES

Fluid Ounces	U.S.	Imperial	Milliliters
	1 teaspoon	1 teaspoon	5
¼	2 teaspoons	1 dessertspoon	10
½	1 tablespoon	1 tablespoon	14
1	2 tablespoons	2 tablespoons	28
2	¼ cup	4 tablespoons	56
4	½ cup		110
5		¼ pint or 1 gill	140
6	¾ cup		170
8	1 cup		225
9			250
10	1¼ cups	½ pint	280
12	1½ cups		340
15		¾ pint	420
16	2 cups		450
18	2¼ cups		500
20	2½ cups	1 pint	560
24	3 cups		675
25		1¼ pints	700
27	3½ cups		750
30	3¾ cups	1½ pints	840
32	4 cups or 1 quart		900
35		1¾ pints	980
36	4½ cups		1000
40	5 cups	2 pints or 1 quart	1120
48	6 cups		1350
50		2½ pints	1400
60	7½ cups	3 pints	1680
64	8 cups or 2 quarts		1800
72	9 cups		2000

OVEN TEMPERATURE EQUIVALENTS

Fahrenheit	Celsius	Gas Mark	Description
225	110	¼	Cool
250	130	½	
275	140	1	Very Slow
300	150	2	
325	170	3	Slow
350	180	4	Moderate
375	190	5	
400	200	6	Moderately Hot
425	220	7	Fairly Hot
450	230	8	Hot
475	240	9	Very Hot
500	250	10	Extremely Hot

EQUIVALENTS FOR INGREDIENTS

all-purpose flour—plain flour
arugula—rocket
confectioners' sugar—icing sugar
cornstarch—cornflour
eggplant—aubergine
granulated sugar—castor sugar
half and half—12% fat milk
lima beans—broad beans
scallion—spring onion
shortening—white fat
squash—courgettes or marrow
unbleached flour—strong, white flour
vanilla bean—vanilla pod
zest—rind
zucchini—courgettes

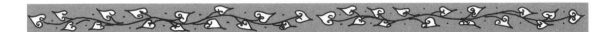
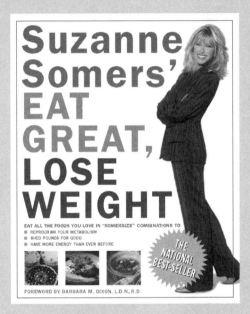
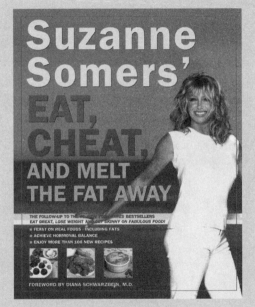

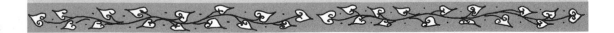